INT-Integrated Neurocognitive Therapy
for Schizophrenia Patients

Volker Roder
Daniel R. Müller
Editors

INT-Integrated Neurocognitive Therapy for Schizophrenia Patients

Springer

Editors
Volker Roder
Professor of Clinical Psychology
University Hospital of Psychiatry and Psychotherapy
University of Bern
Switzerland
roder@sunrise.ch

Daniel R. Müller
Senior Lecturer
University Hospital of Psychiatry and Psychotherapy
University of Bern
Switzerland
daniel.mueller@spk.unibe.ch

Translation of the German edition to English: Aaron Kuchle, South Korea
Translation sponsored by: Hans & Annelies Swierstra Stiftung: www.has-stiftung.ch

Additional material to this book can be downloaded from http://extras.springer.com

ISBN 978-3-319-38205-0 ISBN 978-3-319-13245-7 (eBook)
DOI 10.1007/978-3-319-13245-7

Springer Cham Heidelberg New York Dordrecht London

Softcover reprint of the hardcover 1st edition 2015

Cover illustration by Artur Heras: www.arturheras.com

Printed on acid-free paper

Springer International Publishing AG Switzerland is part of Springer Science+Business Media (www.springer.com)

Preface to the German Edition

Since the turn of the century, international interest in the cognitive treatment of patients with schizophrenia has steadily increased. This is in large part due to the fact that several studies have shown that cognitions are of central importance for coping with life's challenges successfully and for social (re)integration – and thus for the overall life satisfaction of the persons concerned. At the beginning of the 21st century, the NIMH (National Institute of Mental Health) of the USA spearheaded the MATRICS initiative (Measurement and Treatment Research to Improve Cognition in Schizophrenia) with the objective, among others, of consistently defining and measuring cognitions. The initiative's first successes were in the area of neurocognition (e.g., attention, concentration, memory). Yet, there was a growing realization that social cognition (e.g., emotions, social perception processes) is also a crucial factor for persons affected by schizophrenia. As a result, the MATRICS initiative further specified and analyzed the area of social cognition during the end of the first decade of the 21st century. Key exponents of the MATRICS initiative include, among others, the psychologists Michael Green and Keith Nuechterlein of UCLA (University of California, Los Angeles). Associated therapeutic approaches were being conceived at the same time.

The Integrated Psychological Therapy (IPT) program, developed by our team in Bern in the 1980s, was one of the first international therapeutic approaches which, long before the "new wave of cognitive schizophrenia," took into account the significance of cognitions for the treatment of schizophrenia. In the meantime, 37 international studies involving 1,632 patients have proven the success of IPT's implementation. The IPT treatment manual has been translated into 13 languages and is being used in Europe; North, Central, and South America; Asia; and Australia.

About seven years ago, the MATRICS initiative and IPT became the basis for the development of INT. The idea was to develop a therapy approach for patients who were largely socially integrated and in low-threshold treatment, but who suffered from deficits in cognitive functioning. Such patients could not be reached optimally using the cognitive subprograms of IPT, which had been conceived more for patients with pronounced negative symptoms. INT thus systematically converts the areas defined by MATRICS into therapeutic approaches while making use of IPT's empirical results and practical experience in practicing group therapy with persons suffering from schizophrenia.

This treatment manual is divided into six chapters. ▸ Chapter 1 (Theoretical Background) provides an overview of recovery, MATRICS, and IPT that is relevant to the conception of INT. Chapter 2 (Practical Implementation of INT) describes in a highly practical way INT's four treatment areas (A–D) for the improvement of neurocognition and social cognition. This chapter encompasses methods, therapy content, and numerous examples of practical implementation in INT groups. In ▸ Chap. 3 (Therapy Requirements, Possible Applications, and Indication), readers are given concrete information about starting INT groups in their own institutional context. Finally, ▸ Chap. 4 (Diagnostic Instruments, Treatment Planning, and Controlling the Treatment Process) focuses on conceptualizing cases and the significance of INT application. Assessment tools for various functional areas are presented in detail. ▸ Chap. 5 (Empirical Evidence of INT) reports on the results of a multicenter evaluation of INT and critically discusses the relevance of those results for INT practice. Finally, on the ▸ CD-ROM (▸ Chap. 6: Therapy Materials for the Four Treatment Areas), extensive materials are provided for the therapist to print out for distribution. Bibliographical references are listed at the end of each chapter for the interested reader.

The multicenter study (▸ Chap. 5) required about five years to complete – writing and revision of the present volume, nearly one year more. Without the help and support of many people, this work would never have succeeded. We would thus in conclusion like to thank all those who directly or indirectly contributed to the success of this treatment manual: first and foremost of course, all the patients who were willing to try out the many new materials during group sessions, and also all the therapists from the eight centers who implemented INT for the first time in the context of the multicenter evaluation study. These include, in Switzerland, the Psychiatric Hospital of the University of Zürich (A. Theodoridou, M.D.), the Biel Center of Psychiatry (A. Rausch, M.D.), and the University Hospital of Psychiatry and Psychotherapy in Bern; in Germany, the Protestant Hospital of Bielefeld, the Bethel Clinic for Psychiatry and Psychotherapy (M. Driessen, M.D.; C. Barenbrock, M.Sc.), the Rehabilitation Center for the Mentally Ill in Peiting-Herzogsägmühle (S. Queri, Ph.D.; A. Gabrecht, M.D.), ARBEWE Rehabilitation Center in Nuremberg (A. Baumann, M.Sc.; G. Fisher), and the Rehabilitation Center of Vitos Eltville (G. Deutschle, M.Sc.); and in Austria, the State Hospital of Schwarzach/St. Veit (M. Keglevic, M.D.). In addition, we thank our colleagues in Bern who were entrusted with treatment or with diagnostic surveys and data evaluation: Manuela Christen, M.Sc.; Juliane Emmerich, M.Sc.; Annette Eugster, B.Sc.; Lea Hulka, M.Sc.; Stefanie Schmidt, Ph.D.; Daniela Speiser, M.Sc.; and James Weiss, M.Sc. We would like to extend special thanks to our former colleague Marc Lächler, Ph.D., with whom we first elaborated the INT treatment approach. Many thanks also go to Francine Perret, who assisted us in the preparation of various photographs in the materials section.

Last but not least, we would like to extend our thanks to Renate Scheddin, M.D., and Renate Schulz from Springer Publishers, Germany, who showed understanding for delays in manuscript deadlines and always provided us with helpful support.

Volker Roder
Daniel R. Müller
Switzerland

Foreword to the German Edition

The development of Integrated Neurocognitive Therapy (INT) for schizophrenia patients represents the culmination of a long and rich history of comprehensive psychological therapies coming from the group in Bern around Hans Brenner and Volker Roder. I remember well my several visits to Bern for stimulating international conferences focused on the identification and modification of cognitive and social processes in schizophrenia. The Bern tradition has been characterized for many years by sophistication and breadth in conceptualizing the basic psychological and cognitive deficits in schizophrenia. Well before the current scientific acceptance of systematic cognitive remediation as an efficacious intervention for the core cognitive deficits of schizophrenia, the Bern group developed one of the first broad cognitive training approaches, Integrated Psychological Therapy (IPT). IPT is characterized by a series of systematic, manualized modules using group treatment to build skills ranging from basic neurocognition to complex interpersonal problem solving. Through IPT, the Bern group was one of the earliest to integrate treatment of core neurocognitive deficits (e.g., attention, memory, problem solving) with treatment of social cognitive deficits (e.g., social perception, interpersonal problem solving), drawing creatively on the principles of cognitive development, social learning, cognitive behavior therapy, and social skills training. The considerable literature evaluating the efficacy of IPT is impressive and has led to its broad application.

The recent development of INT described here by Volker Roder and Daniel Müller represents a substantial refinement and extension of IPT to incorporate more recent theoretical and empirical advances in the field. One key influence was the NIMH initiative, Measurement and Treatment Research to Improve Cognition in Schizophrenia (MATRICS), inspired by the late Wayne Fenton at NIMH. Through the MATRICS initiative, Michael Green and I led a Neurocognition Committee that surveyed the empirical literature and brought together more than 100 experts to reach consensus on seven key separable cognitive domains in schizophrenia that are fruitful intervention targets – speed of processing, attention/vigilance, working memory, verbal learning, visual learning, reasoning and problem solving, and social cognition. A subsequent related NIMH conference further delineated five key aspects of social cognition – emotional processing, social perception, Theory of Mind, social schema, and attribution style. INT is structured around these separable cognitive domains, moving systematically from initial modules focusing on simpler neurocognitive and social cognitive processes to later modules focusing on high-level integrative neurocognitive and social cognitive processes. Thus, it covers within a single approach a series of training exercises that target all of the cognitive domains identified by the MATRICS initiative.

Another key influence that Roder and Müller have incorporated into INT is the use of computer-based cognitive training, which was not a feature of IPT but has recently become popular in cognitive remediation. Thus, INT includes computerized cognitive remediation as a component of its sessions, increasing the ability to provide multiple practice exercises in focused areas to improve cognitive skills. At the same time, INT retains the distinctive IPT tradition of group treatment sessions, using computerized training as one modality but providing much more group training in social reasoning, strategic planning, and interpersonal problem solving than most current cognitive remediation approaches. INT also emphasizes group processes to enhance engagement in the intervention, including team competition and debates to reach consensus.

A third key feature of INT, relative to most other cognitive remediation approaches, is that it combines restorative and compensatory approaches to the core cognitive and social cognitive deficits in schizophrenia. Other prominent cognitive remediation approaches focus very predominantly on one or the other. INT involves direct exercises to improve cognitive skills to reduce the core deficits, while recognizing that less severe cognitive deficits will nevertheless remain. Thus, participants are helped to identify ways to work around remaining deficits in the context of situations from everyday life, which should further aid the impact of INT on functional outcomes in schizophrenia.

In summary, Roder, Müller, and their colleagues are to be congratulated on the significant advance that INT represents. It retains distinctive features of IPT while incorporating several recent key conceptual and methodological advances. The results of their recent international multisite study of INT show the positive impact that this new comprehensive intervention can achieve. The availability of this volume will hopefully greatly aid the application of INT at additional sites. INT shows excellent promise for improving the cognitive skills and social functioning of patients with schizophrenia, which would be an important step forward for all of us who labor to help those suffering from this disorder.

Keith H. Nuechterlein, Ph.D.
Professor, UCLA Departments of Psychiatry and Biobehavioral Sciences and of Psychology
Co-Chair, MATRICS Neurocognition Committee
Director, Center for Neurocognition and Emotion in Schizophrenia
Director, UCLA Aftercare Research Program

Contents

Theoretical Background

S. J. Schmidt, V. Roder

Additional material (CD-ROM) to this book can be downloaded from http://extras.springer.com

V. Roder, D.R. Müller (eds.), *INT-Integrated Neurocognitive Therapy for Schizophrenia Patients*,
DOI 10.1007/978-3-319-13245-7_1, © Springer International Publishing Switzerland 2015

1.1 "Recovery" and its Effects on the Treatment and Rehabilitation Process

Originally, schizophrenia was viewed as a chronic illness with an irreversibly progressive course (Kraepelin 1913). However, both the recovery movement and empirical findings are working against this stigma of incurability (Zipursky et al. 2013; Strauss 2014; Jääskeläinen et al. 2013). For example, the holistic human approach of the recovery movement stresses overcoming illness-related impairments and leading an autonomous and meaningful existence despite the diagnosis of schizophrenia (Amering and Schmolke 2009). Recovery is now the guideline in health policy in many countries in the area of health promotion and psychiatric care. This is supported by the findings of several long-term clinical studies, which found unexpectedly high recovery rates between 25 and 65 % (Rabinowitz et al. 2007; Davidson et al. 2008). Yet there is still no single, uniform definition of "recovery". The idea of recovery has been influenced by different viewpoints and conceptualized in various ways.

1.1.1 Functional Recovery

In the scientific literature, the concept of recovery is usually based on symptom remission and the re-attainment of a premorbid level of functioning (Nasrallah et al. 2005). An American team headed by Andreasen et al. (2005) was the first to formulate criteria of remission for a schizophrenia disorder. However, these refer solely to a reduction of psychopathological symptoms over a period of 6 months. Yet recovery goes far beyond mere symptom remission, as a person's level of psychosocial functioning is relatively independent of the actual symptoms (Green et al. 2000; Ventura et al. 2010). For instance, a person suffering from schizophrenia might experience psychotic symptoms but nonetheless be able to cope with everyday life. The concept of functional recovery takes this into consideration. It demands, in addition to a sustained reduction of symptoms, the recovery or acquirement of the social skills necessary for an independent existence and thus an adequate level of psychosocial functioning (van Os et al. 2006; Leucht and Lasser 2006; Mausbach et al. 2009; Brekke and Nakagami 2010). Disturbances in psychosocial functioning are central diagnostic criteria for a schizophrenia disorder (DSM-IV; Saß et al. 1994). For example, persons suffering from schizophrenia are less likely to be in a stable relationship, and their social networks are smaller and less supportive. Only 10 to 20 % are employed on a long-term basis in the open labor market. Difficulties also arise in leading an independent life: Tasks such as cooking for oneself, finding a permanent residence, budgeting finances, and taking medication regularly are often impossible without assistance (McGlashan 1988; Häfner 2005; Harvey et al. 2007). These functional disturbances are highly prevalent (Bottlender et al. 2010) and are very stressful for the persons involved as well as their social environment (Bellack et al. 2007). Schizophrenia disorders are thus considered by the World Health Organization to be one of the five most common causes for impairment and invalidity among young adults in industrialized countries (Murray and Lopez 1996). With this in mind, it is of the utmost importance that the factors influencing psychosocial disturbances are identified and modified therapeutically (Harvey et al. 2007). One's level of psychosocial functioning can be considered to be the result of a complex interaction of prior and persisting conditions, conditions which vary in importance intraindividually and interindividually. Neurocognitive and social-cognitive skills represent an important part of these influencing factors (▶ Sect. 1.2). Yet other factors appear to be relevant as well: negative symptoms (Ventura et al. 2009; Rassovsky et al. 2011), social skills and competencies, insight into the illness (Emsley et al. 2008), social support, motivation (Gard et al. 2009), sex, level of premorbid social functioning, age at the start of the illness (Häfner 2005; San et al. 2007), duration of untreated psychosis (Shrivastava et al. 2010), and functional performance (Bowie et al. 2010). Determining the level of psychosocial functioning has remained difficult, since this is a multidimensional construct for which only inconsistent definitions exist so far (Bellack et al. 2007; Leifker et al. 2011). Moreover, the level of psychosocial functioning is influenced by a number of environmental factors such as the amount of financial support, the current situation of the labor market, and the availability of therapy options. It has thus proved advisable to distinguish between the level of performance a person can achieve under optimal conditions (functional performance) and the level he or she exhibits in the real world (Bowie et al. 2006, 2010). This distinction is also being taken into consideration in the current development and evaluation of assessment instruments for the determination of various aspects of psychosocial functioning (Green et al. 2008, 2011; Mausbach et al. 2009; Leifker et al. 2011).

1.1.2 Subjective Recovery

The meaning of "recovery" has also been widened by a movement composed of individuals personally affected by schizophrenia. For them, recovery does not represent an outcome. Rather, it embodies the process of overcoming the personal and social consequences of their illness. The representatives of this movement thus stress that the functional definition of recovery is overly standardized. Such definitions need to take the subjective experiences of the affected persons more into account. These experiences include motivation, self-efficacy, personal responsibility and empowerment, resilience (resistance to crises) as well as insight into one's own resources and impairments (Amering and Schmolke 2009). The self-perception of persons suffering from schizophrenia with respect to their cognitive resources and weaknesses thus often greatly diverges from neuropsychological test results (Medalia et al. 2008). Intrinsic motivation has also proven to be an important factor affecting whether patients profit from a therapy program (Roder et al. 2006).

These two different perspectives of recovery are not mutually exclusive. Rather, they have a dynamically interactive and compensatory relationship. For the treatment and rehabilitation of a person suffering from schizophrenia, this means that therapy should address more than psychosocial impairments. It also should consider the intrinsic motivation and self-efficacy of each and every participant as well as resource activation and the improvement of self-perception as equally important factors. This is only possible if therapy participants see a connection between therapeutic goals and their own objectives and if the therapeutic goals have significance in their daily lives. Regular feedback about their individual progress makes it possible to build up a realistic self-perception of ability, thereby boosting self-efficacy.

Since cognitive functions have proven to be crucial factors affecting the level of psychosocial functioning, they represent an important therapeutic goal of what is currently termed cognitive remediation therapy. These functions will be described in greater detail in the following.

1.2 The Significance of the MATRICS Initiative for Modern Treatment Concepts

For more than three decades now, there has been growing research interest in the cognitive processes of persons with schizophrenia. Experimental psychological research efforts first succeeded in identifying abnormalities in a number of cognitive domains such as elementary visual processing and assessment (Chapman and Chapman 1973; Hemsley 1977; Ruckstuhl 1981). However, the resulting view that cognitive impairments represent pathogenetically significant characteristics has a long tradition, already attracting the interest of Kraepelin (1913) and Bleuler (1911; Palmer et al. 2009). This neuropsychological perspective was also advanced by the conception that schizophrenia is not a neurodegenerative illness but a brain developmental disorder (the "neurodevelopmental model"). According to this interpretation, cognitive deficits reflect prenatally/perinatally acquired or hereditary brain abnormalities of a functional, structural and neurochemical kind. Newly developed, non-invasive methods like functional imaging and neuropsychological tests have made it possible to record these cognitive (dys)functions (Keshavan et al. 2010; Strik et al. 2012). For this reason, we now have at our disposal numerous empirical findings concerning the prevalence and characteristics of cognitive functional deficits and their significance as vulnerability indicators and therapeutic goals. In light of that, the detection of cognitive deficits is now treated as a central criterion in DSM-5 (Barch and Keefe 2010).

Despite mixed study findings, it is today regarded as empirically confirmed that 75 to 85 % of persons diagnosed with schizophrenia exhibit cognitive functional deficits (Gray and Roth 2007; Palmer et al. 2009). This rate of prevalence is even higher if we take the premorbid level of cognitive functioning into account (Goldberg et al. 1990). Meta-analytic studies have reached the conclusion that the average test performance of patients with schizophrenia is at least one standard deviation below that of healthy controls in most cognitive areas (Fioravanti et al. 2005; Dickinson et al. 2007; Mesholam-Gately et al. 2009). The severity of the impairments proved to be relatively independent of the age of the person, duration of hospitalization, clinical symptoms and antipsychotic treatment (Green et al. 2004; Gray and Roth 2007). Current studies suggest a general deficit in information processing. Episodic, declarative memory and processing speed appear to be the most affected. On the other hand, implicit memory and visual-spatial abilities remain relatively intact (Palmer et al. 2009; Kern et al. 2010). In comparison to persons diagnosed with a schizoaffective or bipolar disorder, those suffering from schizophrenia have much lower quantitative test performances. Qualitative differences in test performance or a profile specific to schizophrenia have not yet been identified (Krabbendam et al. 2005; Bora et al. 2009).

Against this background, processes of human information processing have become a central focus as possible vulnerability indicators within explanatory models for the etiology of schizophrenia and thus as intermediary phenotypic markers for the early detection of the illness (Nuechterlein et al. 1994). This is supported by the fact that persons who received a later diagnosis of schizophrenia exhibit cognitive functional deficits already during childhood (Niendam et al. 2003; Osler et al. 2007), during

1

adolescence (Osler et al. 2007) and in the prodromal phase of the condition (Becker et al. 2010; Woodberry et al. 2010; Carrión et al. 2011). Even psychiatrically inconspicuous biological relatives of persons with schizophrenia are impaired at least partially (Keshavan et al. 2010; Eack et al. 2010; Bhojraj et al. 2011). Consistent with the vulnerability hypothesis, there was an increase in the onset of psychosis among persons at risk exhibiting serious cognitive functional deficits (Seidman et al. 2010). The level of cognitive functioning seems to stabilize with respect to the extent of cognitive deficits after the first psychotic episode, at least up to the age of 65. However, certain specific cognitive functions also fluctuate with the psychotic symptoms or recover fully after the initial episode of the illness (Wykes and van der Gaag 2001; Palmer et al. 2009).

Increasing understanding of the importance of cognitions led to the development of several therapeutic strategies and assessment instruments. Disagreement concerning which cognitive domains are relevant and how they can be assessed reliably and validly became an obstacle to the further exploration and evaluation of new therapy programs. With this in mind, the MATRICS initiative (Measurement and Treatment Research to Improve Cognition in Schizophrenia) of the National Institute of Mental Health (NIMH) set out to find a consensus regarding the definition of the most important cognitive domains and, on this basis, to develop a standardized battery of tests. This was meant to accelerate the evaluation of new, at first predominantly pharmacological forms of intervention for the improvement of cognitive impairments (Green and Nuechterlein 2004; Nuechterlein et al. 2004; Kern and Horan 2010). On the basis of expert surveys and factor-analytic studies, six neurocognitive functional areas were identified, all relatively independent of each other (Nuechterlein et al. 2004; Roder et al. 2010, 2011; Table 1.1):

- **Speed of information processing**: This area concerns how quickly information is processed and requires both motor and perceptual abilities.
- **Attention/vigilance**: Selective attention is the ability to select stimuli according to their relevance and to focus on target stimuli while ignoring disturbing stimuli (distractors). On the other hand, vigilance designates the state of maintaining attention over an extended period in situations with a low stimulus frequency.
- **Verbal and visual learning and memory**: These two neurocognitive domains encompass the perception and storage of verbal and nonverbal information. The MATRICS initiative decided on two separate areas for the processing of verbal and visual information because persons with schizophrenia exhibit different impairments in these areas.

Table 1.1 Neurocognitive MATRICS areas

Neurocognitive areas	Description	Impairments
Speed of information processing	Speed of the information to be processed	Less information per unit of time
Attention/ vigilance	Filtering of information Selective attention/ sustained attention (vigilance)	Lack of filtering and suppression of irrelevant stimuli; Longer reaction times, increased distractibility, and lack of reaction to target stimuli
Verbal and visual learning and memory	Intake and storage of verbal and nonverbal information	Impaired learning and recall performance; Relatively intact implicit, procedural memory
Working memory	Verbal, visual, and spatial short-term memory	Lacking maintenance and manipulation of visual-spatial and verbal information
Reasoning and problem solving	Complex strategies for planning and decision-making	Impairments in cognitive flexibility; Deficits in action planning

Nuechterlein et al. (2004), Roder et al. (2010)

- **Working memory**: Working memory has the function of storing verbal and spatial information that is relevant to action. This is constantly adjusted to the current situation, making it possible to control one's behavior in a planned way.
- **Reasoning and problem-solving**: Together with working memory, this area is summarized by the concept of "executive functions". These functions include cognitive flexibility, concept formation, and planning and problem-solving abilities. They also include the ability to monitor one's own actions and to suppress them in favor of new objectives.

The MATRICS initiative first concentrated solely on differentiating neurocognitive areas. Later, the concept of social cognition was developed due to its growing theoretical and practical importance for research and treatment. Social-cognitive processes refer to the processes of information processing upon which social interactions are based. Among these is the ability to interpret the intentions, characteristics, and behaviors of other persons and to react appropriately to them (Brothers 1990; Green et al.

2005, 2008). On the other hand, the area of neurocognition generally includes processes of human information processing (i.e. operations involving the assignment, association, and evaluation of information). These form the basis of human experience and behavior, but relate only to non-social content (Roder et al. 2008). The MATRICS initiative led to the development of a standardized, commercially available battery of tests (MCCB: www.matricsinc.org/MCCB.htm) (Buchanan et al. 2011). So far, it consists of ten measurement tools for recording the six neurocognitive areas and the social-cognitive domains of emotion perception. The MATRICS initiative has further developed the concept of social cognition and currently distinguishes between five social-cognitive areas (Green et al. 2005, 2008; Roder et al. 2010) (► Sect. 1.2; ◘ Table 1.2):

- **Emotion processing**: This area comprises the perception and utilization of emotions. Emotion perception has often been investigated among patients with schizophrenia, typically with the use of facial expressions.
- **Social perception**: This refers to the ability to understand central features of social situations and interactions.
- **Theory of mind (ToM)**: This construct describes the ability mentally to represent the intentions, characteristics, and assumptions of other persons by adopting their perspectives and to make inferences based on these. This is important in order to predict, to explain, or to influence the behavior of others.
- **Social schemata/social knowledge**: Social schemata are knowledge structures in long-term memory. They contain declarative or procedural information about which roles, rules, and goals characterize certain social situations. They are thus crucially involved in the encoding of new information and have an action-guiding function.
- **Social attribution styles**: These include the causal explanations a person generates for particular experiences of success or failure in order to understand social situations and events.

◘ Table 1.2 Social-cognitive MATRICS areas

Social-cognitive areas	Description	Impairments
Emotion perception	Perception and use of emotions	Slower and less accurate recognition of emotional stimuli; Impaired regulation of emotional reactions
Social perception	Recognition and evaluation of social roles and rules in interpersonal situations	Impaired recognition of social cues; Deficient processing of contextual information
Theory of mind (ToM)	Ability to empathize with other people and to infer their intentions	Difficulty understanding false assumptions, deception, irony, metaphors, and cues
Social schemata	Knowledge representations about social norms and roles	Faulty knowledge representations; Impaired access to and/or implementation of this information
Social attributions	Causal attribution following experiences of success or failure	Excessive form of internal attribution for positive events; External attribution in the case of failure ("self-serving bias")

Green et al. (2005), Schmidt et al. (2011)

The social-cognitive processes of persons suffering from schizophrenia have been generating increasing interest since the mid-1990s. However, the history of their research began much earlier (Penn et al. 1997, 2006). In the 1950s and 1960s for example, schizophrenia studies were conducted that concerned the influence of experimental and social contexts on test performance (Cromwell and Spaulding 1978), on the perception of emotional images (Buss and Lang 1965) and on social reasoning processes (Gillis 1969). These papers set crucial foundations, yet it was hardly possible to interpret the results, since the researchers lacked operational definitions of the concepts under investigation and suitable assessment instruments. The reason for the renewed interest in the area of social cognition in schizophrenia research appears above all to be its central role in integrative models for the level of psychosocial functioning and for recovery (◘ Fig. 1.1).

According to this model, the level of psychosocial functioning of a person with schizophrenia is determined by multiple factors: neurocognitive and social-cognitive functions, positive and negative symptoms, and the orientation of the treatment. Cross-sectional and longitudinal empirical studies were able to confirm the relationship postulated in the model between neurocognitive areas and the level of psychosocial functioning (Green et al. 2000, 2004; Milev et al. 2005; Bowie et al. 2006; Cohen et al. 2006; Brekke and Nakagami 2010). The percentage of explained variance of the level of psychosocial functioning ranged between 20 and 40 % (Couture et al. 2006). As a result, 60–80 % of the variance in the level of psychosocial

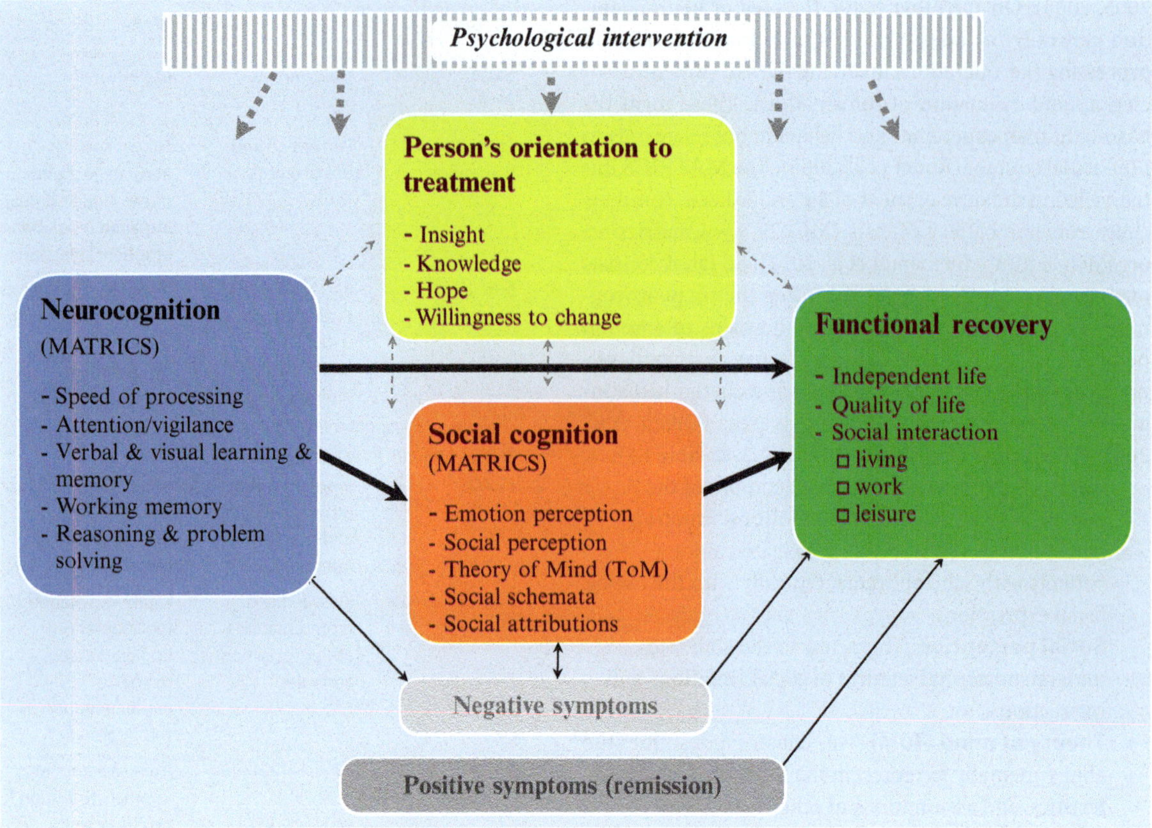

Fig. 1.1 Integrative model: possible mediators between cognitions and functional recovery (Roder et al. 2010)

functioning could not be explained by performance differences in the neurocognitive test. This prompted the search for further influential factors and for an answer to the question of how these relationships originate. Social-cognitive functions became a point of central focus because they exhibit consistent associations with neurocognitive areas (Brüne et al. 2007) and are considered to be essential determinants of the level of psychosocial functioning (Couture et al. 2006; Fett et al. 2011). Although neurocognition and social cognition are interconnected constructs, there is empirical evidence that they are not redundant:

- The correlations are only of average magnitude (Wykes and Reeder 2005).
- A neural network appears to exist that is specialized in the processing of social information (Brunet-Gouet and Decety 2006; Pinkham et al. 2008).
- Differential impairments in neurocognitive or social-cognitive functions are possible (Pinkham et al. 2003).
- After monitoring the influence of neurocognitive functions, social-cognitive functions explain an additional amount of variance of the level of psychosocial functioning (Addington et al. 2006; Pinkham and Penn 2006).

Current studies have found evidence that the correlation between basal neurocognitive functions and the level of psychosocial functioning in patients with schizophrenia is mediated by social-cognitive functions. In other words, social-cognitive functions act as a mediator variable in this correlation (Schmidt et al. 2011). The area of negative symptoms is being discussed as a further mediator variable (Ventura et al. 2009; Couture et al. 2011; Rassovsky et al. 2011). In studies, at least moderate correlations were found between neurocognitive and social-cognitive areas and that of negative symptoms. The question of causality remains unexplained to this day, but study results suggest that cognitive impairments are more the cause than the effect of negative symptoms (Bowie and Harvey 2005; Kirkpatrick et al. 2006; Sergi et al. 2007). In longitudinal studies, changes in negative symptoms proved to be relatively independent of cognitive changes and yielded differential correlations with the level of psychosocial functioning, which also speaks for a separation of these areas (Bowie et al. 2010; Foussias and Remington 2010). The extent of positive symptoms on the other hand had fewer correlations with cognitive functions and the level of psychosocial functioning than did the negative symptoms. However, some parameters do appear to fluctuate with acute psychotic episodes. During remission, these parameters seem also to be associated with an improvement of function recovery (Wykes and van der Gaag 2001; Bertrand et al. 2007; Ventura et al. 2010).

The recovery concept also stresses the significance of the patient's individual treatment orientation for therapy responsiveness. This includes the patient's insight into his or her problems as well as knowledge of the disorder and how to cope with it. Other influential factors that appear to be especially decisive for therapeutic success include motivation (Medalia and Lim 2004; Velligan et al. 2006; Gard et al. 2009; Choi and Medalia 2010), empowerment/self-efficacy as well as hope and knowledge (Resnick et al. 2005; Sibitz et al. 2011).

This integrative model (Fig. 1.1) makes it clear that approaches to psychological therapy from each of these areas can apply neurocognitive and social-cognitive remediation therapy, cognitive-behavioral therapy for the treatment of persisting positive symptoms, therapy of social competencies or psychoeducation, and family therapy (Roder et al. 2010). Because of the great number of factors influencing the level of psychosocial functioning, integrative approaches that embed cognitive and social factors into a multimodal therapeutic concept appear to be especially promising. Therefore, our definition of an integrative neurocognitive approach encompasses two aspects: An intervention is integrative if, in addition to neurocognitive functions, at least one of the following areas is therapeutically impacted: social cognition, knowledge about the illness/difficulties/resources, social skills in the residential, vocational, and recreational domains, and cognitive thought patterns (e.g. irrational beliefs). Moreover, the term "integrative" makes it clear that therapy should always be based on a multimodal treatment concept, individual rehabilitation goals, and the cognitive resources and weaknesses of each participant.

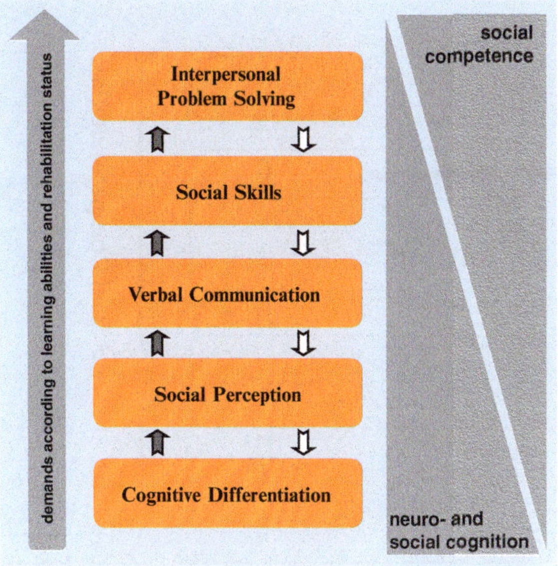

Fig. 1.2 Integrated Psychological Therapy (IPT) – contents and therapy concept (Roder et al. 2008, 2010; with kind permission of Beltz Verlag)

1.3 Further Developments of Integrated Psychological Therapy (IPT): INT and WAF

One example of such an integrated neurocognitive therapy program is Integrated Psychological Therapy (IPT) (Roder et al. 1988, 2008, 2010). It combines neurocognitive and social-cognitive remediation therapy with the therapy of social competencies and interpersonal problem-solving abilities. IPT is divided into five modules of increasing complexity which build upon each other (Fig. 1.2): In the first module, "Cognitive Differentiation", various neurocognitive functions should be improved (e.g. attention, verbal memory, cognitive flexibility, concept-formation). The second module, "Social Perception", addresses operations of social-cognitive information processing such as social and emotional perception. The link between the first two cognitively oriented modules and the last two, more behavior-oriented modules is established by the third module, "Verbal Communication". It aims at improving verbal fluency and executive functions, which are necessary for interpersonal relationships. In the last two modules, "Social Skills" and "Interpersonal Problem Solving", role play and group problem-solving exercises promote the acquisition of social skills. The group is led by one therapist and one co-therapist and comprises five to eight participants. It is best carried out twice a week for 60 min over a period of at least 3 months. Additional homework assignments, in vivo exercises, and individual therapy supplement these group sessions.

IPT has been evaluated in 36 independently published studies in 12 countries in Europe, America and Asia (Roder et al. 2006, 2011). The manual is now obtainable in 13 languages. The summarization of these individual study results in meta-analytic techniques speaks for the effectiveness of IPT in comparison to placebo-attention or empty control groups in the area of neurocognition and

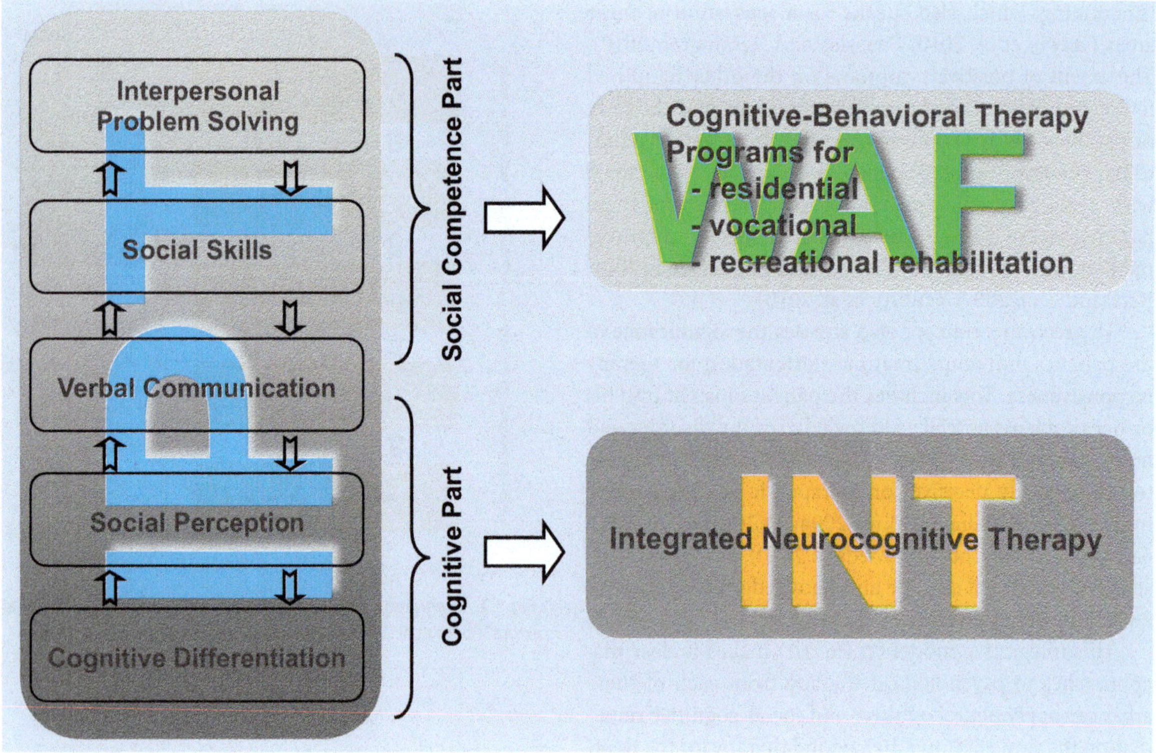

Fig. 1.3 Further developments of Integrated Psychological Therapy (IPT) (Roder et al. 2008, 2010; with kind permission of Beltz Verlag)

social cognition, negative symptomatology, and the level of psychosocial functioning. These effects also remained unchanged after a follow-up period (Roder et al. 2006, 2010). IPT thus represents one of the first systematic, manual-based cognitive approaches to group therapy for people suffering from schizophrenia. IPT was initially conceived over 30 years ago (Brenner et al. 1980). IPT's conception thus anticipated the growing importance of social cognition and an integrative approach to treatment. On the basis of the IPT approach, two further developments arose against the backdrop of the new state of empirical and theoretical knowledge described above (Fig. 1.3).

As an initial step, our team expanded the two IPT modules "social skills" and "interpersonal problem solving" by developing specific group therapy programs for social competencies in the residential, vocational, and recreational domains (abbreviated WAF, from the German "Wohnen, Arbeit, Freizeit") (Roder et al. 2008). WAF has the aim of sensitizing participants' perceptions of their own needs in these areas of everyday life. Building upon this, it strives to support the formation of goals for specific residential, vocational, or recreational situations. In order to help implement patients' decisions, the group rehearses necessary social competencies and activates both potential difficulties and existing resources. WAF too has been evaluated in effectiveness studies. These showed, in conformity with the recovery perspective, that the therapy's concern with everyday life contributed to an increase in patient motivation. This is a decisive prerequisite for improving social competencies and reducing negative symptoms (Mueller and Roder 2005; Roder et al. 2006).

Integrated Neurocognitive Therapy (INT) represents a further step in this development. IPT also had an influence on INT's treatment approach and therapeutic methods. INT encompasses all 11 of the neurocognitive and social-cognitive MATRICS areas and thus expands on the first two IPT modules. The combined treatment of neurocognitive and social-cognitive functions are also based on the results of IPT research: Implementation of all five IPT modules resulted, with the same therapy duration, in greater and longer-lasting effects compared with individual neurocognitive modules (Roder et al. 2006, 2010; Mueller et al. 2007). IPT focuses initially on basal neurocognitive functions before moving increasingly to social-cognitive processes and finally to complex interpersonal skills. This didactic structure makes it possible for the participants to become accustomed to the group context quickly. They can also have a sense of achievement already at the beginning of the therapy process thanks to clearly structured tasks which are not emotionally stressful. Improvement of basal neurocognitive functions appears to be a necessary requirement for the rehabilitation of social-cognitive functions and social skills, since they are seen to be limiting factors for therapy success. Accordingly, the therapeutic content of INT is also organized into sequential modules. In the process of therapy, the degree of emotional activation and the complexity of the exercises grow with time while being increasingly less structured by the therapists. Consistent with IPT, INT was also conceived as a cognitive-behavioral approach to group therapy. The reason for this is that, in this setting, group processes arise that are relevant to everyday life but nonetheless provide safe conditions, thus easing the learning of social skills (Mueller et al. 2011).

Given the theoretical background outlined here and the current state of empirical knowledge, an integrative and well-coordinated treatment and rehabilitation of patients with schizophrenia from the standpoints of both functional and subjective recovery remains an important future goal. Studies have showed that medicinal treatment with typical and atypical neuroleptics yield few positive effects on the level of cognitive functioning, with moderate effects on negative symptoms and the level of psychosocial functioning (Bowie and Harvey 2005; Harvey et al. 2007; Keefe et al. 2007, 2011). Accordingly, the importance of multidimensional, integrative approaches to psychological treatment, focusing on the cognitive and social impairments brought on by the illness, will increase considerably in the years ahead.

References

Addington, J., Saeedi, H., & Addington, D. (2006). Facial affect recognition: A mediator between cognitive and social functioning in psychosis. *Schizophrenia Research, 85*(1–3), 142–150.

Amering, M., & Schmolke, M. (2009). *Recovery in mental health. Reshaping scientific and clinical responsibilities*. London: Wiley-Blackwell.

Andreasen, N. C., Carpenter, W. T. J., Kane, J. M., Lasser, R. A., Marder, S. R., & Weinberger, D. R. (2005). Remission in schizophrenia: Proposed criteria and rationale for consensus. *American Journal of Psychiatry, 162*, 441–449.

Barch, D. M., & Keefe, R. S. (2010). Anticipating DSM-V: Opportunities and challenges for cognition and psychosis. *Schizophrenia Bulletin, 36*(1), 43–47.

Becker, H. E., Nieman, D. H., Wiltink, S., Dingemans, P. M., van de Fliert, L., van Amelsvoort, T. A., & Linszen, D. H. (2010). Neurocognitive functioning before and after the first psychotic episode: Does psychosis result in cognitive deterioration? *Psychological Medicine, 40*, 1599–1606.

Bellack, A. S., Green, M. F., Cook, J. A., Fenton, W., Harvey, P. W., Heaton, R. K., Laughren, T., Leon, A. C., Mayo, D. J., Patrick, D. L., Patterson, T. L., Rose, A., Stover, E., & Wykes, T. (2007). Assessment of community functioning in people with schizophrenia and other severe mental illnesses: A white paper based on an NIMH-sponsored workshop. *Schizophrenia Bulletin, 33*, 805–822.

Bertrand, M. C., Sutton, H., Achim, A. M., Malla, A. K., & Lepage, M. (2007). Social cognitive impairments in first episode psychosis. *Schizophrenia Research, 95*, 124–133.

Bhojraj, T., Francis, A., Montrose, D. M., & Keshavan, M. S. (2011). Grey matter and cognitive deficits in young relatives of schizophrenia patients. *NeuroImage, 54*(1), 287–92.

Bleuler, E. (1911). *Dementia Praecox oder die Gruppe der Schizophrenien*. Leipzig: Deuticke.

Bora, E., Yucel, M., & Pantelis, C. (2009). Cognitive endophenotypes of bipolar disorder: A meta-analysis of neuropsychological deficits in euthymic patients and their first-degree relatives. *Journal of Affective Disorders, 113*, 1–20.

Bottlender, R., Strauß, A., & Möller, H.-J. (2010). Social disability in schizophrenic, schizoaffective and affective disorders 15 years after admission. *Schizophrenia Research, 116*, 9–15.

Bowie, C. R., & Harvey, P. D. (2005). Cognition in schizophrenia: Impairments, determinants, and functional importance. *Psychiatric Clinics of North America, 28*, 613–633.

Bowie, C. R., Reichenberg, A., Patterson, T. L., Heaton, B. K., & Havey, P. D. (2006). Determinants of real-world functional performance in schizophrenia subjects: Correlations with cognition, functional capacity, and symptoms. *American Journal of Psychiatry, 163*, 418–425.

Bowie, C. R., Depp, C., McGrath, J. A., Wolyniec, P., Mausbach, B. T., Thornquist, M. H., Luke, J., Patterson, T. L., Harvey, P. D., & Pulver, A. E. (2010). Prediction of real-world functional disability in chronic mental disorders: A comparison of schizophrenia and bipolar disorder. *American Journal of Psychiatry, 167*(9), 116–1124.

Brekke, J., & Nakagami, E. (2010). The relevance of neurocognition and social cognition for outcome and recovery in schizophrenia. In V. Roder & A. Medalia (Eds.), *Neurocognition and social cognition in schizophrenia patients Comprehension and treatment* (pp. 23–36). Basel: Karger.

Brenner, H. D., Stramke, W. G., Mewes, J., Liese, F., & Seeger, G. (1980). Erfahrungen mit einem spezifischen Therapieprogramm zum Training kognitiver und kommunikativer Fahigkeiten in der Rehabilitation chronisch schizophrener Patienten. *Nervenarzt, 51*, 106–112.

Brothers, L. (1990). The social brain: A project for integrating primate behavior and neurophysiology in a new domain. *Concepts in Neuroscience, 1*, 27–51.

Brüne, M., Abdel-Hamid, M., Lehmkämper, C., & Sonntag, C. (2007). Mental state attribution, neurocognitive functioning, and psychopathology: What predicts poor social competence in schizophrenia best? *Schizophrenia Research, 92*(1–3), 151–159.

Brunet-Gouet, E., & Decety, J. (2006). Social brain dysfunctions in schizophrenia: A review of neuroimaging studies. *Psychiatry Research, 148*(2–3), 75–92.

Buchanan, R. W., Keefe, R. S., Umbricht, D., Green, M. F., Laughren, T., & Marder, S. R. (2011). The FDA-NIMH-MATRICS guidelines for clinical trial design of cognitive-enhancing drugs: what do we know 5 years later? *Schizophrenia Bulletin, 37*(6), 1209–17.

Buss, A., & Lang, P. (1965). Psychological deficit in schizophrenia: Affect reinforcement and concept attainment. *Journal of Abnormal Psychology, 70*, 2–24.

Carrión, R. E., Goldberg, T. E., McLaughlin, D., Auther, A. M., Correll, C., & Cornblatt, B. A. (2011). Impact of neurocognition on social and role functioning in individuals at clinical high risk for psychosis. *American Journal of Psychiatry, AiA*, 1–8.

Chapman, L. J., & Chapman, J. P. (1973). *Disordered thought in schizophrenia*. Englewood Cliffs: Prentice Hall.

Choi, J., & Medalia, A. (2010). Intrinsic motivation and learning in a schizophrenia spectrum sample. *Schizophrenia Research, 118*, 12–19.

Cohen, A. S., Forbes, C. B., Mann, M. C., & Blanchard, J. J. (2006). Specific cognitive deficits and differential domains of social functioning in schizophrenia. *Schizophrenia Research, 81*, 227–238.

Couture, S. M., Penn, D. L., & Roberts, D. L. (2006). The functional significance of social cognition in schizophrenia: A review. *Schizophrenia Bulletin, 32*, 44–63.

Couture, S. M., Granholm, E. L., & Fish, S. C. (2011). A path model investigation of neurocognition, theory of mind, social competence, negative symptoms and real-world functioning in schizophrenia. *Schizophrenia Research, 125*(2–3), 152–160.

Cromwell, R. L., & Spaulding, W. (1978). How schizophrenics handle information. In W. E. Fann, I. Karacan, A. D. Pokorny, & R. L. Williams (Eds.), *The phenomenology and treatment of schizophrenia* (pp. 127–162). New York: Spectrum.

Davidson, L., Schmutte, T., Dinzeo, T., & Andres-Hyman, R. (2008). Remission and recovery in schizophrenia: Practitioner and patient perspectives. *Schizophrenia Bulletin, 34*, 5–8.

Dickinson, D., Ramsey, M. E., & Gold, J. M. (2007). Overlooking the obvious: A meta-analytic comparison of digit symbol coding tasks and other cognitive measures in schizophrenia. *Archives of General Psychiatry, 64*, 532–542.

Eack, S. M., Mermon, D. E., Montrose, D. M., Miewal, J., Gur, R. E., Gur, R. C., Sweeney, J. A., & Keshavan, M. S. (2010). Social cognition deficits among individuals at familial high risk for schizophrenia. *Schizophrenia Bulletin, 36*(6), 1081–8.

Emsley, R., Oosthuizen, P., Koen, L., Niehaus, D., Medori, R., & Rabinowitz, J. (2008). Remission in patients with first-episode schizophrenia receiving assured antipsychotic medication: A study with risperidone long-acting injection. *International Clinical Psychopharmacology, 23*(6), 325–331.

Fett, A. K., Viechtbauer, W., Dominguez, M. D., Penn, D. L., van Os, J., et al. (2011). The relationship between neurocognition and social cognition with functional outcomes in schizophrenia: A meta-analysis. *Neuroscience and Biobehavioral Review, 35*, 573–588.

Fioravanti, M., Carlone, O., Vitale, B., Cinti, M. E., & Clare, L. (2005). A meta-analysis of cognitive deficits in adults with a diagnosis of schizophrenia. *Neuropsychology Review, 15*, 73–95.

Foussias, G., & Remington, G. (2010). Negative symptoms in schizophrenia: avolition and Occam's razor. *Schizophrenia Bulletin, 36*(2), 359–69.

Gard, D. E., Fisher, M., Garrett, C., Genevsky, A., & Vinogradov, S. (2009). Motivation and its relationship to neurocognition, social cognition, and functional outcome in schizophrenia. *Schizophrenia Research, 115*, 74–81.

Gillis, J. S. (1969). Schizophrenic thinking in a probabilistic situation. *Psychological Record, 19*, 211–224.

Goldberg, T. E., Berman, K. F., Mohr, E., & Weinberger, D. R. (1990). Regional cerebral blood flow and cognitive function in Huntington's disease and schizophrenia: A comparison of patients matched for performance on a prefrontal-type task. *Archives of Neurology, 47*, 418–422.

Gray, J. A., & Roth, B. L. (2007). Molecular targets for treating cognitive dysfunction in schizophrenia. *Schizophrenia Bulletin, 33*, 1100–1119.

Green, M. F., & Nuechterlein, K. H. (2004). The MATRICS initiative: Developing a consensus cognitive battery for clinical trials. *Schizophrenia Research, 72*, 1–3.

Green, M. F., Kern, R. S., Braf, D. L., & Mintz, J. (2000). Neurocognitive deficits and functional outcome in schizophrenia: Are we measuring the "Right Stuff"? *Schizophrenia Bulletin, 26*(1), 119–136.

Green, M. F., Kern, R. S., & Heaton, R. K. (2004). Longitudinal studies of cognition and functional outcome in schizophrenia: Implications for MATRICS. *Schizophrenia Research, 72*(1), 41–51.

Green, M. F., Olivier, B., Crawley, J. N., Penn, D. L., & Silverstein, S. (2005). Social cognition in schizophrenia: Recommendations from the measurement and treatment research to improve cognition in schizophrenia new approaches conference. *Schizophrenia Research, 31*, 882–887.

Green, M. F., Nuechterlein, K. H., Kern, R. S., Baade, L. E., Fenton, W. S., Gold, J. M., Keefe, R. S. E., Mesholam-Gately, R., Seidman, L. J., Stover, E., & Marder, S. R. (2008). Functional co-primary measures for clinical trials in schizophrenia: Results from the MATRICS psychometric and standardization study. *American Journal of Psychiatry, 165*(2), 221–228.

Green, M. F., Schooler, M. R., Kern, R. S., Frese, F. J., Granberry, W., Harvey, P. D., Karson, C. N., Peters, N., Stewart, M., Seidman, L. J., Sonnenberg, J., Stone, W. S., Walling, D., Stover, E., & Marder, S. R. (2011). Evaluation of functionally meaningful measures for clinical trials of cognition enhancement in schizophrenia. *American Journal of Psychiatry, 168*, 400–407.

Häfner, H. (2005). *Das Rätsel Schizophrenie – Eine Krankheit wird entschlüsselt, 3. vollständig überarbeitete Auflage.* München: Beck.

Harvey, P. D., Velligan, D. I., & Bellack, A. S. (2007). Performance-based measures of functional skills: Usefulness in clinical treatment studies. *Schizophrenia Bulletin, 33*(5), 1138–1148.

Hemsley, D. R. (1977). What have cognitive deficits to do with schizophrenic symptoms? *British Journal of Psychiatry, 130*, 167–173.

Jääskeläinen, E., Juola, P., & Hirvonen, N. (2013). A systematic and meta-analysis of recovery in schizophrenia. *Schizophrenia Bulletin, 39*(6), 1296–1306.

Keefe, R. S. E., Bilder, R. M., Davis, S. M., Harvey, P. D., Palmer, B. W., Gold, J. M., Meltzer, H. Y., Green, M. F., et al. (2007). Neurocognitive effects of antipsychotic medications in patients with chronic schizophrenia in the CATIE trial. *Archives of General Psychiatry, 64*, 633–647.

Keefe, R. S. E., Fox, K. H., Harvey, P. D., Cuchiaro, J., Siu, C., & Loebel, A. (2011). Characteristics of the MATRICS consensus cognitive battery in a 29-site antiphlogistic schizophrenia clinical trial. *Schizophrenia Research, 125*(2–3), 161–168.

Kern, R. S., & Horan, W. P. (2010). Definition and measurement of neurocognition and social cognition. In A. Medalia & V. Roder (Eds.), *Neurocognition and social cognition in schizophrenia patients. Comprehension and treatment.* Karger: Basel.

Kern, R. S., Hartzell, A. M., Izaguirre, B., & Hamilton, A. H. (2010). Declarative and non-declarative memory in schizophrenia: What is impaired? What is spared? *Journal of Clinical and Experimental Neuropsychology, 32*, 1017–1027.

Keshavan, M. S., Kulkarni, S., Bhojraj, T., Francis, A., Diwadkar, V., Montrose, D. M., Seidman, L. J., & Sweeney, J. (2010). Premorbid cognitive deficits in young relatives of schizophrenia patients. *Frontiers in Human Neuroscience, 3*(62), 1–14.

Kirkpatrick, B., Fenton, W., Carpenter, W. T., & Marder, S. R. (2006). The NIMH-MATRICS consensus statement on negative symptoms. *Schizophrenia Bulletin, 32*, 296–303.

Krabbendam, L., Myin-Germeys, I., Bak, M., & Van Os, J. (2005). Explaining transitions over the hypothesized psychosis continuum. *Australian and New Zealand Journal of Psychiatry, 39*, 180–186.

Kraepelin, E. (1913). *Psychiatrie. Ein Lehrbuch für Studierende und Ärzte. 3. Band: Klinische Psychiatrie, 2. Teil.* Leipzig: Barth.

Leifker, F. R., Patterson, T. L., Heaton, R. K., & Harvey, P. D. (2011). Validating measures of real-world outcome: The results of the VALERO expert survey and RAND panel. *Schizophrenia Bulletin, 37*(2), 334–343.

Leucht, S., & Lasser, R. (2006). The concepts of remission and recovery in schizophrenia. *Pharmacopsychiatry, 39*, 161–170.

Mausbach, B. T., Moore, R., Bowie, C., Cardenas, V., & Patterson, T. L. (2009). A review of instruments for measuring functional recovery in those diagnosed with psychosis. *Schizophrenia Bulletin, 35*(2), 307–318.

McGlashan, T. H. (1988). A selective review of recent North American long-term followup studies of schizophrenia. *Schizophrenia Bulletin, 14*(4), 515–542.

Medalia, A., & Lim, R. W. (2004). Self-awareness of cognitive functioning in schizophrenia. *Schizophrenia Research, 71*, 331–338.

Medalia, A., Thysen, J., & Freilich, B. (2008). Do people with schizophrenia who have objective cognitive impairments identify cognitive deficits on a self-report measure? *Schizophrenia Research, 105*, 156–164.

Mesholam-Gately, R. I., Giuliano, A. J., Goff, K. P., Faraone, S. V., & Seidman, L. J. (2009). Neurocognition in first-episode schizophrenia: A meta-analytic review. *Neuropsychology, 23*, 315–336.

Milev, P., Ho, B. C., Arndt, S., & Andreasen, N. C. (2005). Predictive values of neurocognition and negative symptoms on functional outcome in schizophrenia: a longitudinal first-episode study with 7-year follow-up. *American Journal of Psychiatry, 162*, 495–506.

Mueller, D. R., & Roder, V. (2005). Social skills training in recreational rehabilitation of schizophrenia patients. *American Journal of Recreation Therapy, 4*(3), 11–19.

Mueller, D. R., Roder, V., & Brenner, H. D. (2007). Effektivität des Integrierten Psychologischen Therapieprogramms (IPT). Eine Meta-Analyse über 28 unabhängige Studien. *Nervenarzt, 78*(1), 62–73.

Mueller, D. R., Schmidt, S. J., & Roder, V. (2011). Integrated neurocognitive therapy (INT). In D. L. Penn & D. Roberts (Eds.), *Social cognition in schizophrenia*. New York: Elsevier.

Murray, C. J. L., & Lopez, A. D. (1996). Evidence-based health policy: Lessons from the global burden of disease study. *Science, 274*(5288), 740–743.

Nasrallah, H. A., Targum, S. D., Tandon, R., McCombs, J. S., & Ross, R. (2005). Defining and measuring clinical effectiveness in the treatment of schizophrenia. *Psychiatric Services, 56*, 273–282.

Niendam, T. A., Bearden, C. E., Rosso, I. M., Sanchez, L. E., Hadley, T., Nuechterlein, K. H., & Cannon, T. D. (2003). A prospective study of childhood neurocognitive functioning in schizophrenic patients and their siblings. *American Journal of Psychiatry, 160*(11), 2060–2062.

Nuechterlein, K. H., Dawson, M. E., & Green, M. F. (1994). Information-processing abnormalities as neuropsychological vulnerability indicators for schizophrenia. *Acta Psychiatrica Scandinavica/Supplementum, 384*, 71–79.

Nuechterlein, K. H., Barch, D. M., Gold, J. M., Goldberg, T. E., Green, M. F., & Heaton, T. E. (2004). Identification of separable cognitive factors in schizophrenia. *Schizophrenia Research, 72*, 29–39.

Osler, M., Lawlor, D. A., & Nordentoft, M. (2007). Cognitive function in childhood and early adulthood and hospital admission for schizophrenia and bipolar disorders in Danish men born in 1953. *Schizophrenia Research, 92*(1–3), 132–141.

Palmer, B. W., Dawes, S. E., & Heaton, R. K. (2009). What do we know about neuropsychological aspects of schizophrenia? *Neuropsychology Review, 19*(3), 365–384.

Penn, D. L., Corrigan, P. W., Bentall, R. P., Racenstein, J. M., & Newman, L. (1997). Social cognition in schizophrenia. *Psychological Bulletin, 121*(1), 114–132.

Penn, D. L., Addington, J., & Pinkham, A. (2006). Social cognitive impairments. In J. A. Lieberman, T. S. Stroup, & D. O. Perkins (Eds.), *The American psychiatric publishing textbook of schizophrenia* (pp. 261–274). London/Washington, DC: American Psychiatric Publishing, Inc.

Pinkham, A. E., & Penn, D. L. (2006). Neurocognitive and social cognitive predictors of interpersonal skill in schizophrenia. *Psychiatry Research, 143*, 167–178.

Pinkham, A. E., Penn, D. L., Perkins, D. O., & Lieberman, J. (2003). Implications for the neural basis of social cognition for the study of schizophrenia. *American Journal of Psychiatry, 160*(5), 815–824.

Pinkham, A. E., Hopfinger, J. B., Pelphrey, K. A., Piven, J., & Penn, D. L. (2008). Neural bases for impaired social cognition in schizophrenia and autism spectrum disorders. *Schizophrenia Research, 99*(1–3), 164–175.

Rabinowitz, J., Levine, S. Z., Haim, R., & Häfner, H. (2007). The course of schizophrenia: Progressive deterioration, amelioration or both? *Schizophrenia Research, 91*, 254–258.

Rassovsky, Y., Horan, W. P., Lee, J., Sergi, M. J., & Green, M. F. (2011). Pathways between early visual processing and functional outcome in schizophrenia. *Psychological Medicine, 41*, 487–497.

Resnick, S., Fontana, A., Lehman, A. F., & Rosenheck, R. (2005). An empirical conceptualization of the recovery orientation. *Schizophrenia Research, 75*, 119–128.

Roder, V., Brenner, H. D., Kienzle, N., & Hodel, B. (1988). *Integriertes Psychologisches Therapieprogramm (IPT) für schizophrene Patienten*. Weinheim: Psychologie Verlags Union.

Roder, V., Mueller, D. R., Mueser, K. T., & Brenner, H. D. (2006). Integrated Psychological Therapy (IPT) for schizophrenia: Is it effective? *Schizophrenia Bulletin, 32*(1), 81–93.

Roder, V., Brenner, H. D., & Kienzle, N. (2008). *Integriertes Psychologisches Therapieprogramm bei schizophren Erkrankten IPT*. Weinheim: Beltz.

Roder, V., Mueller, D. R., Brenner, H. D., & Spaulding, W. (2010). *Integrated psychological therapy (IPT) for the treatment of neurocognition, social cognition and social competency in schizophrenia patients*. Göttingen, Seattle: Hogrefe and Huber.

Roder, V., Mueller, D. R., & Schmidt, S. J. (2011). Effectiveness of integrated psychological therapy (INT) for schizophrenia patients: A research update. *Schizophrenia Bulletin, 37*(2), 71–79.

Ruckstuhl, U. (1981). *Schizophrenieforschung*. Beltz: Weinheim.

San, L., Ciudad, A., Alvarez, E., Bobes, J., & Gilaberte, I. (2007). Symptomatic remission and social/vocational functioning in outpatients with schizophrenia: Prevalence and associations in a cross-sectional study. *European Psychiatry, 22*, 490–498.

Saß, H., Wittchen, H.-and, & Zaudig, M. (Hrsg.) (1994). *Diagnostisches und Statistisches Manual Psychischer Störungen (DSM-IV)*. Göttingen: Hogrefe.

Schmidt, S., Mueller, D. R., & Roder, V. (2011). Social cognition as a mediator variable between neurocognition and functional outcome in schizophrenia: Empirical review and new results by structural equation modeling. *Schizophrenia Bulletin, 37*(2), 41–54.

Seidman, L. J., Giuliano, A. J., Meyer, E. C., Addington, J., Cadenhead, K. S., Cannon, T. D., Mcglashan, T. H., Perkins, D. O., Tsuang, M. T., Walker, E. F., Woods, S. W., Bearden, C. E., Christensen, B. K., Hawkins, K., Heaton, R., Keefe, R. S., Heinssen, R., & Cornblatt, B. A. (2010). Neuropsychology of the prodrome to psychosis in the NAPLS consortium: Relationship to family history and conversion to psychosis. *Archives of General Psychiatry, 67*, 578–588.

Sergi, M. J., Rassovsky, Y., Widmark, C., Reist, C., Erhart, S., Braff, D. L., Marder, S. R., & Green, M. F. (2007). Social cognition in schizophrenia: Relationships with neurocognition and negative symptoms. *Schizophrenia Research, 90*, 316–324.

Shrivastava, A., Johnston, M., Shah, N., & Bureau, Y. (2010). Redefining outcome measures in schizophrenia: Integrating social and clinical parameters. *Current Opinion in Psychiatry, 23*, 120–126.

Sibitz, I., Amering, M., Unger, A., Seyringer, M. E., Bachmann, A., Schrank, B., Benesch, T., Schulze, B., & Woppmann, A. (2011). The impact of the social network, stigma and empowerment on the quality of life in patients with schizophrenia. *European Psychiatry, 26*(1), 28–33.

Strauss, J. (2014). Reconceptualizing schizophrenia. *Schizophrenia Bulletin, 40*(suppl. 2), S97–S100.

Strik, W., Schmidt, S. J., & Roder, V. (2012). Cognition and schizophrenia. In S. Pallanti & J. Lauriello (Eds.), *Clinical manual of schizophrenia*. Arlington: American Psychiatric Publishing.

van Os, J., Burns, T., Cavallaro, R., Leucht, S., Peuskens, J., Helldin, L., Bernardo, M., Arango, C., Fleischhacker, W., Lachaux, B., & Kane, J. M. (2006). Standardized remission criteria in schizophrenia. *Acta Psychiatrica Scandinavica, 113*, 91–95.

Velligan, D. I., Kern, R. S., & Gold, J. M. (2006). Cognitive rehabilitation for schizophrenia and the putative role of motivation and expectancies. *Schizophrenia Bulletin, 32*, 474–485.

Ventura, J., Hellemann, G. S., Thames, A. D., Koellner, V., & Nuechterlein, K. H. (2009). Symptoms as mediators of the relationship between neurocognition and functional outcome in schizophrenia. *Schizophrenia Research, 113*, 189–199.

Ventura, J., Reise, S. P., Keefe, R., Baade, L. E., Gold, J. M., Green, M. F., Kern, R. S., Mesholam-Gately, R., Nuechterlein, K. H., Seidman, L. J., & Bilder, R. M. (2010). The cognitive assessment interview (CAI): Development and validation of an empirically derived, brief interview-based measure of cognition. *Schizophrenia Research, 121*, 24–31.

Woodberry, K. A., Seidman, L. J., Giuliano, A. J., Verdi, M. B., Cook, W. L., & McFarlane, W. R. (2010). Neuropsychological profiles in individuals at clinical high risk for psychosis: Relationship to psychosis and intelligence. *Schizophrenia Research, 123*, 188–198.

Wykes, T., & Reeder, C. (2005). *Cognitive remediation therapy for schizophrenia*. London/New York: Routledge.

Wykes, T., & van der Gaag, M. (2001). Is it time to develop a new cognitive therapy for psychosis cognitive remediation therapy (CRT)? *Clinical Psychology Review, 21*(8), 1227–1256.

Zipursky, R. B., Reilly, T. J., & Murray, R. M. (2013). The myth of schizophrenia as a progressive brain disease. *Schizophrenia Bulletin, 39*(6), 1363–1372.

Practical Implementation of INT

D. R. Müller, S. J. Schmidt, M. Lächler, V. Roder

Additional material (CD-ROM) to this book can be downloaded from http://extras.springer.com

V. Roder, D.R. Müller (eds.), *INT-Integrated Neurocognitive Therapy for Schizophrenia Patients*,
DOI 10.1007/978-3-319-13245-7_2, © Springer International Publishing Switzerland 2015

The purpose of this chapter is to provide information about the practical implementation of Integrated Neurocognitive Therapy (INT) in the light of our clinical experience. Building upon the theoretical and empirical background (▶ Chap. 1), we will first introduce INT's therapeutic approach. The individual areas of treatment (modules), use of therapy materials, didactic structure, and the infrastructural requirements for implementation will be explained in a practice-oriented way by means of examples. The user can become gradually acquainted with the therapeutic interventions and follow the 30 example sessions. The sections closing the chapter address aspects of motivation building, forming relationships, and group processes that are central for INT and for group therapy in general.

2.1 Overview, Structure, and Didactics of Integrated Neurocognitive Therapy

2.1.1 Therapeutic Approach

INT's therapeutic strategy is based on that of IPT (Roder et al. 2008a, 2010). It follows a hierarchical model that integrates the various function and symptom areas relevant to schizophrenia into a comprehensive approach (◘ Fig. 1.1). In this approach to schizophrenia treatment, functional recovery (or successful coping with everyday life) is seen as the highest stage of functionality and the top rehabilitation goal. This is achieved when the patient can shape his or her life more independently, has an improved quality of life, and is better integrated socially. Neurocognitive and social-cognitive impairments determine the success of such rehabilitation, as do resources, negative symptoms, and treatment orientation.

Being a group therapy approach, INT makes use of group processes and group dynamics in each module (therapy area). At the same time, treatment is always focused on the individual cognitive deficits and resources of the patients. INT is thus equivalent to a resource-oriented approach to group therapy with a wide intervention spectrum and broad intervention goals.

2.1.2 Therapeutic Goals

INT's therapeutic goals follow from the integrative recovery model introduced in ▶ Chap. 1 (◘ Fig. 1.1):

Neurocognition One basic goal is the improvement of the neurocognitive functions defined by the MATRICS initiative (Green & Nuechterlein 2004, Nuechterlein et al. 2004) (◘ Table 1.1). This lays the foundation for further rehabilitation since neurocognitive limitations can prevent further therapy success. INT is thus a neurocognitive approach to remediation therapy.

Social Cognition A second basic goal of INT is to improve the social-cognitive functions specified by the MATRICS initiative (Green et al. 2005) (◘ Table 1.2). By addressing social-cognitive functionality, we can thus integrate not only the social context into the therapeutic process but also emotional and interpersonal stress. Furthermore, consistent use of group resources and group dynamics promotes social cognition throughout the course of treatment. INT thus represents a social-cognitive approach to remediation therapy as well.

Finally, INT also aims to improve mediating factors from the area of treatment orientation.

Insight INT encourages insight into problems associated with cognitive deficits and resources that arise regularly in the everyday life of a person with schizophrenia. The creation of an individual cognitive profile promotes a more realistic estimation of one's own level of functioning in various cognitive functional areas. With this patient group, self-assessment of cognitive capabilities frequently does not agree with objective test results (Medalia and Thysen 2008). For this reason, INT constantly aims to integrate the patient's insight into her own cognitive capabilities into the intervention process.

Knowledge Successful improvement of insight goes hand in hand with educating the patient about the disorder and ways of coping with it. INT differs in this respect from conventional psychoeducational programs. The educative process focuses not on the schizophrenia disorder itself but rather on cognitive functions. Accordingly, the interventions are not geared towards coping with (positive) symptoms, but towards compensating for cognitive deficits and optimizing cognitive resources.

Motivation Greater insight and knowledge concerning one's own cognitive capabilities also boosts the INT participant's intrinsic motivation. Persons suffering from schizophrenia often show little motivation in therapy, making successful treatment difficult. Intrinsic motivation is thus an effective, nonspecific mechanism of action in psychotherapeutic treatment (Barch and Carter 2005; Velligan et al. 2006; Nakagami et al. 2008). For this reason, INT pays particular attention to improving and maintaining motivation (▶ Sect. 2.5).

Expectation of Self-Efficacy Another of INT's intervention goals is to improve the patient's expectation of self-efficacy.

Establishing the expectation of being able to achieve something on one's own is an important factor for any psychotherapeutic intervention. INT consistently integrates the everyday life of the patients into the group therapy process. It attempts to make improvement strategies experienceable for the patients, particularly in group exercises. Successful experiences of coping with problems and of using their own resources help patients become aware that they can achieve things independently.

Functional Recovery (▶ Chap. 1) and Negative Symptoms
These are not direct intervention goals in INT. Yet our long-term experience with IPT has shown that integrated neurocognitive and social-cognitive remediation therapy can also help improve the level of psychosocial functioning and reduce negative symptoms (Roder et al. 2010, 2011; Müller and Roder 2008). Thus, one secondary goal of INT is to lay the foundation for the (re-)establishment of social skills by improving neurocognitive and social-cognitive functions.

Summary of Therapeutic Goals
- Improvement of neurocognitive functions as the foundation for further therapeutic steps: speed of information processing, attention and vigilance, verbal and visual learning and memory, reasoning and problem solving, working memory (MATRICS)
- Improvement of social-cognitive functions: emotional processes, social perception, theory of mind (ToM), social schemas, and social attributions (MATRICS)
- Promotion of insight, knowledge, motivation, expectation of self-efficacy
- Reduction of negative symptoms as a secondary treatment goal
- Improvement of the level of psychosocial functioning as a secondary treatment goal

2.1.3 Therapy Components

In INT, the six neurocognitive and five social-cognitive functional areas defined by the MATRICS initiative are integrated into a single therapeutic framework. To each cognitive functional area are assigned corresponding cognitive/behavioral exercises. The 11 cognitive functional areas are organized into four areas of treatment (modules). Each area of treatment begins with a neurocognitive section, followed by a social-cognitive section. ◻ Figure 2.1 shows a diagram of the four INT modules.

The sequence of the four treatment areas was established using the following criteria:

- Increase in the level of difficulty of therapy content
- Increase in the emotional stress caused by therapy content
- Gradual reduction of the amount of therapeutic structuring in the course of treatment

In other words: INT begins with less complex and affectively non-emphasized neurocognitive content in a highly structured group setting and ends with complex, potentially emotional stressful content in interactive exercises in a less structured environment.

The schematic diagram of INT also clarifies the characteristics of a bottom-up and top-down approach: the subject matter of the largely basic first module is implicitly addressed again in the more complex modules following it. In this way, previously handled intervention areas are reinforced by the effect of positive feedback.

2.1.4 Didactic Structure of the INT Modules

Each of the four treatment areas starts with a neurocognitive section. Only then does the social-cognitive section of that module begins, alternating with further neurocognitive exercises. All four INT modules and each intervention unit for all 11 neurocognitive and social-cognitive functional areas within these treatment areas follow the same didactic structure. This structure comprises two therapy components: introductory sessions and follow-up sessions. The follow-up sessions are further subdivided into the components of compensation, restitution, and in vivo exercises/independent exercises. ◻ Table 2.1 provides an overview of INT's didactic structure with the individual therapy components:

▪ Introductory Sessions

Each intervention unit for the 11 cognitive MATRICS functional areas starts with an introduction. The purpose of the introduction is to increase and standardize participant knowledge. The introductory sessions also promote self-perception of everyday resources and difficulties. INT focuses not only on cognitive functional deficits, but also on individual cognitive strengths (resources). Pointing out (new) possibilities of coping with everyday difficulties by using of one's own resources helps build up motivation, especially when supported by a complimentary relationship with the therapist. In addition, patients assess the difficulty of the exercises individually, which also promotes motivation. Possible key questions for the individual assessment of exercises include:

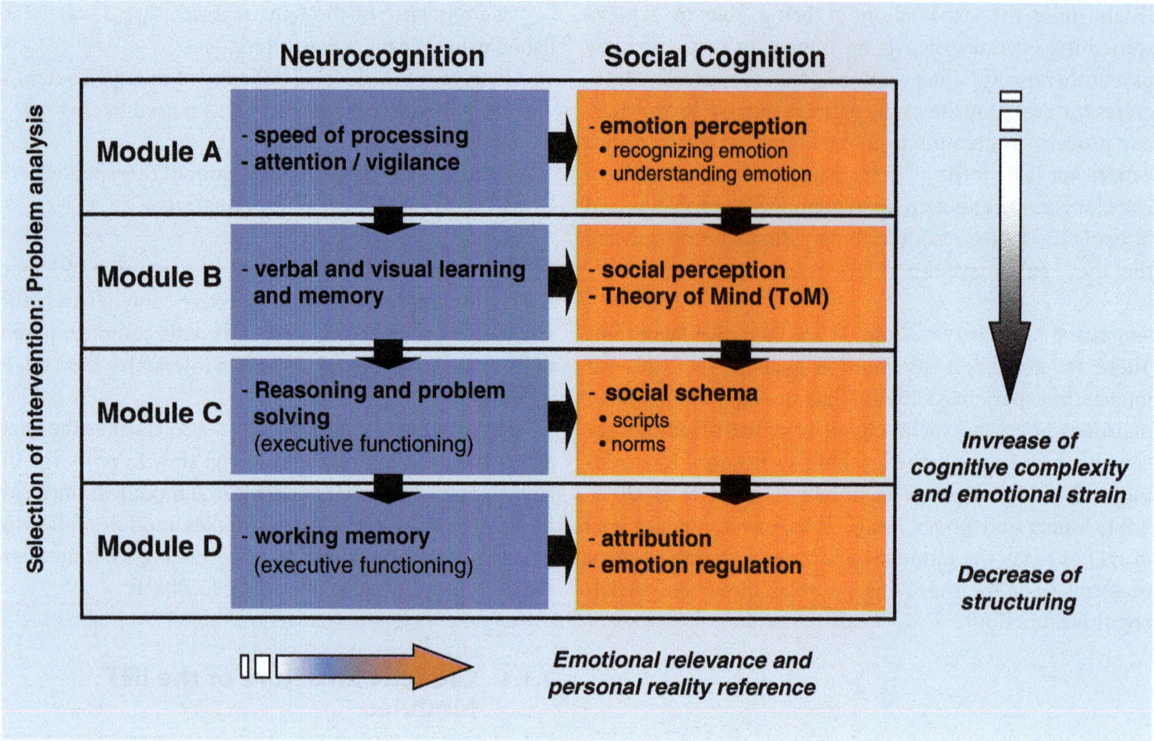

Fig. 2.1 Diagram of INT (Roder et al. 2008a; with kind permission of Beltz Verlag)

Table 2.1 Therapy components and therapy materials of the four INT modules

Therapy components	Materials
Introductory session	
Self-perception of the subjective experience of resources and deficits and optimization possibilities in everyday life	Case vignettes
Education specific to the treatment area for improving insight into problems/ resources and deficits	Information sheets
	Worksheets
Follow-up sessions	
Compensation: The development of coping strategies and interactive application in a group setting	Worksheets
	Information sheets
	Film materials
Restitution: Repeated practice, also using computer-based exercises according to the principle of "errorless learning" in order to habituate learned skills	Written cards
	Depicted stimuli
	Computer program
In vivo exercises: Encouraging transference to everyday life and generalization to other functional areas	Worksheets

Examples of Key Questions

- Did I find the exercise easy?
- Was the exercise fun?
- Why?

or

- Did I find the exercise hard?
- Was it too difficult?
- Did I not like the exercise?

Various therapy materials are available, such as case vignettes, information sheets, and worksheets (▶ Sect. 2.1.5). In addition, it is possible in the neurocognitive section of each module to do a computer-based exercise after introducing the basic topic. The experiences the patients make there of their own deficits and resources can then be used as a starting point for further group elaboration of the cognitive functional area. Clearly structured and easily comprehensible computer exercises have the advantage of being largely free of social stress, so that even patients with pronounced negative symptoms are enabled. Another advantage is the possibility of comparing the results before and after the implementation of compensation strategies. Yet it should be kept in mind that less capable patients often cannot immediately implement compensation strategies they have learned. In order to avoid negative experiences, it is advisable only to compare results that have been improved by repeated practice (habituation) with those of the introductory sessions. It is therefore the responsibility of the therapist to judge how appropriate this method might be in the introductory sessions.

To sum up, the goal of the introductory sessions is that the patients know which basic cognitive skills will be focused on in the next sessions, how they experience these skills in their everyday lives, and how they try – if at all – to avoid related difficulties. It is also important that patients become aware of their own cognitive capabilities in everyday, practical situations. Moreover, encouraging motivation and the ability to change is of central importance in this phase of therapy, as it is essential in order to guarantee active group participation when developing new coping strategies. Again, particular emphasis is placed on discussing the participants' resources in the respective functional areas, as this is especially necessary when beginning treatment with a patient with schizophrenia (▶ Sect. 2.5). As a rule, an emphasis on resources helps ensure relationship-forming and motivation.

▪ Follow-Up Sessions

After the introductory sessions, INT follow-up sessions include various therapy components for each area-specific intervention: a compensation component, a restitution component, in vivo exercises, and independent exercises

▪▪ Compensation

Personal strategies for coping with cognitive deficits in everyday life have already been compiled in the introductory sessions. These sessions also encouraged a positive frame of mind oriented towards solving these problems. Building on this, the group now looks for further coping strategies and supplements existing approaches. These coping strategies must always be concretely formulated and relevant to everyday activities. The second step is to adapt the (now summarized and documented) coping strategies to the individual person. Each group participant assesses which coping strategy is right for him/her and which strategies seem applicable. Using a problem-solving model, individual advantages and disadvantages are discussed, and feared difficulties are anticipated. Finally, the participants try out the new coping strategies in interactive exercises. The regular use of role play in this intervention component supports the implicit learning of the patients. Such interactive exercises make it possible for the patients to have their first experiences with applying learned strategies in a reality-simulating environment. Feedback and discussions with other group members also promote self-reflection about one's own conduct. In the process, the patients are encouraged to employ arguments supported by facts and to avoid assumptions and suspicions. Ongoing motivation-building, positive reinforcement, coaching on the basis of actual coping experiences – all are prerequisites for ensuring active patient participation and for improving expectations of self-efficacy. The goal of INT's compensation component is that the patients trust themselves to actively apply the coping skills they have learned. The therapy materials available for this will be described in detail in the next section.

▪▪ Restitution

The term "restitution" designates the recovery of a function by practice. This repeated practice follows the principle of "practice makes perfect". With this learning principle, it is possible to make demonstrable improvements in the cognitive functioning of patients with schizophrenia in the trained areas. However, the criticism often arises that associated improvements are not stable after completion of the treatment. INT differs in this respect from other classic cognitive remediation approaches. In the latter, a patient often has to solve abstract problems with increasing difficulty and speed, usually without assistance. INT's restitution component is primarily focused on the practical rehearsal of coping strategies for various tasks. One approach to strategy learning is used in the process. New strategies are consolidated and made automatic by repeated practice. Another difference from conventional training is that about half of the INT exercises take place in a group setting, where the focus is on connecting back to everyday life. For example, exercises for improving vigilance are put in the context of the participants' places of work, with all their specific demands and difficulties. In INT, participants work at computers separately or in groups for a maximum of 30 min. After this amount of time, concentration usually declines steadily, even with stable outpatients. To sum up, the overriding goal of INT's restitution component is the repeated application and consolidation of new coping strategies.

▪▪ In Vivo Exercises and Independent Exercises

Finally, each intervention unit concludes with in vivo exercises and independent exercises. If possible, the group accompanies the individual participant during in vivo exercises in real situations. In addition, patients apply coping strategies, which have already been individualized and rehearsed in the group, in independent exercises within their actual social environment. The next group session then starts with a detailed debriefing with regard to the exercise's level of success, emotional stress, conditions specific to the situation, and existing/feared difficulties in the application of coping strategies. The goal is to support the patients' application of newly learned coping strategies in their everyday lives.

2

2.1.5 Therapy Materials

This therapy manual contains an ample amount of therapy materials (on the attached ▶ CD-ROM) for each of the four treatment areas. These are listed separately in ▶ Chap. 6 and can be found on the ▶ CD-ROM. ◘ Table 2.1 provides an overview of the different types of materials used. The following types of therapy materials are employed in INT's educational introductory sections and compensatory sections:

Case Vignettes Representative short stories are available to help introduce the topic of a specific treatment area. These short narratives describe individual cognitive deficits and resources using the everyday experiences of the protagonist, who is named Peter. Group reading and discussion of the short stories introduce the patients to the topic without directly invoking the often stressful, emotionally charged everyday lives of the patients themselves. The group discusses Peter's experiences, not their own. Only later do the patients report on their own everyday experiences. These may coincide with or differ from those described in the short story.

Information Sheets These contain information about therapy content for the purpose of optimizing and standardizing the knowledge of the participants. They also include summaries of possible strategies for coping with cognitive deficits. These coping strategies can be individually supplemented by exploring their particular relevance to each group participant's everyday life.

Worksheets Worksheets contain definitions of terms and explanatory models of cognitive functions and their relevance to everyday life. They serve as the foundation for both group exercises and independent exercises. Worksheets promote the active participation of the patients. They also help individualize general information: patients document the cognitive difficulties they have experienced in concrete, everyday situations and reflect on the success of their application. Goals discussed in the group and the success of their application are also recorded on worksheets. Vignettes, information sheets, and worksheets are all included on ▶ CD-ROM.

Standardized Written Cards Words, sentences, and short texts written on cards serve as language-based stimuli for group exercises. The practical part of this manual (▶ Sect. 2.3) contains specific and detailed instructions on the use of written cards in each exercise. These therapy materials are also on ▶ CD-ROM.

Visual Stimuli The social-cognitive sections of the four INT modules contain a wealth of visually depicted stimuli, all of which are included in PDF format on ▶ CD-ROM. These can be projected (▶ CD e-Materials) or printed out (▶ CD Materials). In addition, the treatment also utilizes cards printed with various designs (card-sorting exercise) as used in the first IPT module (Roder et al. 1988, 2008a, 2010). This interactive card-sorting task for the targeted promotion of group processes is available on paper. Furthermore, the set of pictures of facial affects created by Paul Eckman represent valuable visual stimuli for INT (Ekman and Friesen 1976).

Film Material In the social-cognitive part of the INT modules, selections from commercially available films are also utilized. For copyright reasons, these films have to be acquired by the users themselves. Films that have hitherto proved effective in INT groups are listed in the practical manual sections (▶ Sect. 2.3).

Computer Program A computer program is available for the neurocognitive intervention section of the four INT modules. INT uses the CogPack program distributed by the Marker Software company (Olbrich 1996, 1998, 1999). Due to license reasons, this program is not included in the manual and should be acquired by the users themselves (www.markersoftware.com). CogPack provides exercises for all six neurocognitive MATRICS dimensions. Each exercise follows the principle of "errorless learning" (Kern et al. 2002, 2003, 2005): in order to avoid patient error as much as possible during the exercise, it always begins with the simplest difficulty level and only moves to the next level when 80–90 % of the tasks have been solved correctly. This has the goal of minimizing errors, which can be experienced as emotionally stressful. It also promotes an individualized, automatic response to newly learned skills. After each individual task is completed, the CogPack program provides immediate performance feedback (is the solution right or wrong, what would have been the right answer, completion speed, etc.). This direct program feedback is therapeutically useful for promoting realistic self-perception and self-evaluation of capabilities in the target area. Practical descriptions of independent and group CogPack exercises can be found in ▶ Sect. 2.3.

2.2 Therapeutic Infrastructure

2.2.1 General Conditions

INT group implementation is subject to several general conditions. Particular institutional conditions, a differential indication for participation in INT, risks of group formation, and therapist requirements will be described in detail later in ▶ Chap. 3. We will focus here on general conditions. Before patient recruitment can even begin, infrastructural clarifications must first be made with respect to

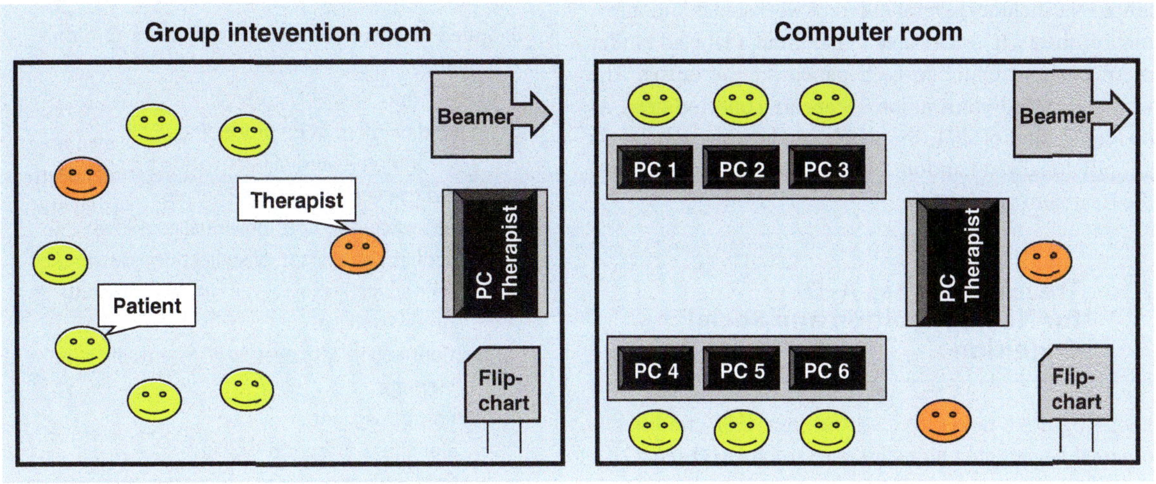

Fig. 2.2 Required materials and rooms (Müller and Roder 2010; with kind permission of Karger Publishers)

available rooms. Also, equipment such as computers, computer programs, projectors, and treatment materials may also need to be organized or acquired.

Room Conditions INT involves group exercises and computer-based exercises. Accordingly, group sessions take place both in a standard group room (preferably with circular or semicircular seating) and in a nearby computer room. In the computer room, one computer with keyboard and mouse is required for each patient and the primary therapist. The standard therapy room should also be equipped with a computer (Fig. 2.2). INT sessions generally take 90 min with an additional break. Within one session, we recommend that no longer than 30 min be spent uninterrupted at a computer. After that, patient concentration and motivation abate markedly. Accordingly, the group switches back and forth between the therapy room and the computer room at least once in the course of a therapy session.

Computers Computer-requirements are modest insofar as the program used, CogPack (▶ Sect. 2.1.5), can be installed with systems using Windows 95. Other computer-based therapy materials are in PDF format. Older, fairly obsolete computers are usually sufficient.

Computer Programs CogPack is distributed by Marker Software. Further information, also about obtaining a user license, is available on the company's homepage: www.markersoftware.com.

Projectors Group exercises involve the use of an ample amount of visually depicted stimuli and film excerpts. These are projected on a screen by a computer with a digital projector. Both the group room and the computer room should have a projector. Alternately, a projector can be transported back and forth between the two rooms.

Flip Charts In group interactions and discussions, the flip chart is an indispensable aid for compiling discussion contributions clearly. Furthermore, it is possible to update therapy content recorded there once again at a later time.

Therapy and Group Materials All therapy materials can be found, with three exceptions, on the enclosed ▶ CD-ROM.

- For copyright reasons, we cannot include commercially distributed films, scenes from which are used for therapeutic purposes. These films have to be obtained by the therapists themselves. A list of films that have proved effective can be found in ▶ Sect. 2.3 (Description of the Four INT Modules).
- The second exception are the tried-and-tested cards printed with four different designs (IPT card-sorting exercise) and the series of pictures for social perception from the Integrated Psychological Therapy program (IPT, 1st and 2nd modules; Roder et al. 1988, 2002, 2008a, 2010). The easily distinguishable designs of the IPT card-sorting exercise vary in the colors, shapes, numbers, and days of the week depicted on them. A set consists of 230 different cards. IPT's two standardized series of pictures for social perception each contain 40 standardized pictures (degree of complexity, emotional stress, basic emotion depicted, etc.). These IPT materials can be obtained from the author (roder@sunrise.ch).
- The Pictures of Facial Affect (PFA) compiled and standardized by Ekman and Friesen (1976) are also not included. Each of the 110 electronically available black-and-white photographs represents either one basic emotion or a lack of affective expression (© Paul Ekman 1993). This visual material can be obtained on the Internet (www.paulekman.com).

Since INT includes several different worksheets and information sheets, it is advisable to hand out a labeled binder or transparent folder to each patient at the outset. The worksheets and information sheets are collected here. At the conclusion of INT, the whole binder then represents an individualized handout, which can be used even after the treatment is over.

2.3 Treatment Areas A–D for Neurocognition and Social Cognition

Each cognitive target area of the four INT modules is organized using the same didactic structure (Table 2.1). Introductory sessions contain area-specific instruction with the specific intention of promoting self-perception of cognitive resources and deficits. Follow-up sessions begin with a compensation component, which is followed by a restitution component. Finally, participants perform in vivo exercises/independent exercises. The various intervention techniques employed will now be described in detail for the intervention components of Module A. For the subsequent modules (B-D), the reader will find only short descriptions with references to Module A.

2.3.1 INT Module A

Module A aims to intervene in two neurocognitive target areas: speed of information processing and attention/vigilance. In the introductory sessions, the first topic is speed of information processing, which is put in connection with attention activation (alertness). The target area of attention and vigilance (concentration) is then introduced. In the ensuing compensation and restitution components, the two neurocognitive target areas are handled together owing to overlapping content. In addition, Module A provides the patients with a general introduction to INT as well as a framework for them to become acquainted with each other.

2.3.1.1 Neurocognitive Intervention Area: Speed of Information Processing and Attention/Vigilance

Module A: Neurocognitive Intervention Area: Speed of Information Processing and Attention/Vigilance

I. Overview of therapy content and getting acquainted
- Getting acquainted
- Establishing group rules

II. Speed of information processing and attention/vigilance

1. Introduction
   - Speed of information processing
     - Definition: speed of information processing
     - Self-perception in the target area
     - Resource-oriented, individual cognitive profile: comparison of subjective assessment with objective test results in computer and group exercises
     - Connection with everyday life and self: case vignette
   - Attention/vigilance
     - Definition: attention/vigilance
     - Self-perception in the target area: overarching theme: understimulation
     - Reference to everyday life and self: case vignette
     - Factors influencing performance: alertness, medication, interests and motivation, mood, daily rhythm (education concerning homogenization of knowledge)
2. Compensation
   - Learning and individualizing coping strategies: speed of information processing and attention/vigilance
   - Coping strategies for maintaining vigilance
   - Area-specific coping strategies:
     - Recreation
     - Difficulties in reading
     - Quality of sleep and lifestyle
     - Vocation
     - Concept-formation: mood and concentration
3. Restitution
   - Habituation of learned coping strategies:
     - Repetition of computer exercises
     - Repetition of group exercises
4. In vivo exercises and independent exercises
   - Transfer of individualized coping strategies to concrete, everyday situations

I. Overview of Therapy Content and Getting Acquainted

Tips

- Infrastructure: group therapy room, flip chart
- Therapy materials: ▶ CD Information Sheet 1
- Didactics: highly structured group discussion

Therapy Content

The patients are informed about the content of the therapy, the materials and formats used, and the organization and sequence of the sessions. This information should be kept concise to avoid overtaxing the patients. An example of a short introduction to INT is found on ► CD Information Sheet 1 on the enclosed ► CD-ROM. Additions made by participants or therapists should also be noted on ► CD Information Sheet 1. As a rule, there are always patients who want to know what INT actually means. If this has not already been explained with each patient in the individual admission interview, therapists should briefly explain the concept of INT using simple language and avoiding technical terms.

Introduction Example

INT stands for Integrated Neurocognitive Therapy. The term "cognitive" stands for different functions that are important for thinking. The term "neuro" means the relationship of these mental functions to the brain. The brain is where mental functions like memory ("I'm trying to remember something") take place. Finally, the term "integrated" has to do with combining, discussing, and exercising the various mental functions within the therapy program, since different mental functions influence each other.

In groups with outpatients and day-care patients, stigmatization experienced by persons suffering from schizophrenia is often a topic of discussion. For this reasons, we use the neutral terms "course" and "(course) participant" instead of "(psycho)therapy group" and "patient".

Getting Acquainted

In an ice-breaking round, the participants and the team of therapists introduce each other. Also, the therapists inquire about the patients' experiences and expectations concerning group therapy and compile them neutrally. Every experienced therapist has their own preferred method in such ice-breaking sessions. Let us use the ball method as an example. The primary therapist throws a ball to a patient and asks: "May I ask what your name is? I'd also like to know about your hobbies and interests." The participant answers this, throws the ball to another participant, and asks the same questions. This procedure is appropriate for uniform groups with mild symptoms and average to high performance levels. With other group configurations, a highly structured process is preferable. In this case, the therapists might ask the participants questions one by one. Such questions could include: "I'd also like to know what you expect from this course", or "Is there something in particular you are afraid of?"

Establishing Group Rules

Group rules concerning the formal workflow of the treatment sessions must also be defined. The following group rules have previously been tried and tested in INT groups. However, they can also be supplemented with other rules introduced by the therapists or the group.

Group Rules

- **No obligation to speak:** Each participant is allowed the possibility of taking a time out (and telling the therapist this) and of being passive during an exercise (i.e., attending without active participation).
- **Mistakes are allowed:** The group should be established as a protected space where mistakes are expressly permitted during exercises. We learn from our mistakes.
- **Mutual support:** Participants mutually support each other; only relevant, constructive criticism is allowed, not personal reproaches.
- **Self-imposed participant discretion:** Participants' ideas and personal contributions are not to be communicated outside the group, but remain in the group room.
- ......

This formal introduction to group therapy is especially important in the psychotherapeutic treatment of patients with schizophrenia. It has the following goals: building up a sustainable group relationship between the participants, forming a supportive, complementary relationship with the therapists, supporting therapy motivation, and creating an atmosphere that is as anxiety-free as possible. This allows the patients to engage themselves with the group and the subject matter.

II. Speed of Information Processing and Attention/Vigilance

Tips

- Infrastructure: group therapy and computer rooms, flip chart, digital projector
- Therapy materials: ► CD Information Sheets 2–5, ► CD Worksheets 1–5, ► CD Vignettes 1–3
- Card-sorting exercises: IPT (► CD Materials 1), speed (► CD Materials 2a–l), concentration and alertness (► CD Materials 3a–b)
- CogPack: speed: VISUMOTOR, UFOs, FALLINGSTARS, BALL, STOP, REACTION
- Attention/vigilance: PIECE-WORK, SEQUENCE, SCAN
- Didactics: highly structured group discussions, individual computer exercises

2.3.1.1.1 Introductory Sessions

2.3.1.1.1.1 Speed of Information Processing

- **Definition of the Target Area: Speed of Information Processing**

The concept of the neurocognitive function "speed of information processing" is described in an introductory way using simple, easily comprehensive language.

Speed is defined as our individual pace in the intake and processing of information and in the resulting reaction.

Examples from everyday life are used for clarification:
- How quickly do I take care of my everyday tasks?
- How quickly do I understand what someone else says to me?
- How quickly do I react when a traffic light changes from red to green?
- How quickly can I work or read? etc.

Concerning the processing of recreational or vocational tasks, the distinction is already made between "accuracy" (attention, concentration) and "speed":
- Those who work very quickly, or even hastily, are more prone to error.
- On the other hand, those who work very precisely and exactly are slower as a result, but probably make fewer errors.

- **Promoting Self-Perception in the Cognitive Target Area**

After this, the participants take turns reporting on how they subjectively assess their own speed as defined above and which situations they see their performance as weak or strong. Their statements are recorded on the flip chart. In addition, each participant receives ► CD Worksheet 1 ("How fast am I?"). Only the questions on that sheet are answered at this point. There are also two questions on the worksheet concerning comparison with others ("I am generally faster than others") and satisfaction ("I am satisfied with my speed"). These questions are an opportunity to address social components and the subjective evaluation of performance, both of which are decisive stress factors. The group discusses the questions on the worksheet to extend self-perception to these topic areas. At this point, ► CD Worksheet 1 serves only as a first stocktaking of individual self-assessment. The connection to patients' everyday lives is later deepened when they have their first experiences with the computer exercises and discuss the case vignettes.

In addition to instructing the participants about the specific topic, the sessions introducing speed of information processing also serve to build up group motivation and cohesion. Factors that should be taken into consideration include potentially inflated mistrust due to persisting positive symptoms, reduced interest and level of activation caused by negative symptoms, and individual participants' inexperience with groups, which can induce anxiety. Depending on the composition of the group, it is advisable not to divulge assessments from the worksheets of participants who exhibit excessive mistrust. Instead, the content should be discussed generally using statistics without specifying concrete assessments.

- **Computer Exercises**

In the introduction to information processing speed, participants already move between the group and computer rooms. This is an exception to INT's general didactic approach when introducing a new cognitive intervention unit. It is done for three reasons:
- The participants are introduced to the CogPack program and learn its operation. Basic computer knowledge is taught, helping inexperienced participants become less anxious dealing with computers.
- CogPack's simple, highly structured and goal-oriented exercises help reduce anxiety-ridden expectations of being in a group in a way that is relatively free of social and emotional stress.
- Objective, immediately reported test results can be compared with previously recorded subjective assessments of patient capabilities in the cognitive target area.

The following CogPack exercises have proved effective: The VISUMOTOR exercise is especially suitable for showing participants how to use the program and the computer mouse. The ease of the exercise helps reduce the fears of inexperienced participants. The exercises UFOs, FALLINGSTARS, or BALL are also recommended, as they are designed as games and tend to activate participants and promote motivation. These and other exercises will be described in detail in the restitution section below. The program's direct feedback after each exercise (e.g., improvements in the second half compared to the first half of the exercise, or improvements in the second round compared to the first based on comparative values) is a key element for promoting adequate self-perception. From a psychotherapeutic point of view, giving the participants positive reinforcement for their test performances is also indispensible. For example, patients should receive praise and acknowledgment simply for engaging in the exercises and carrying them through to the end. If they have difficulties processing the exercises or experience stress, therapists support the patients and help solve the exercise to avoid overstraining them.

After this computer exercise, which is usually kept short, participants then return to the group room. Self-perception is promoted by briefly reflecting on individual experiences. Therapists should register the participants' experiences in an approving and encouraging way.

Questions are discussed such as: "Did I find myself fast or slow?", "Did I try to be as fast as possible?", "What was easy for me?", "Where did I have difficulties?" Patients are generally apt to make self-assessments at this point ("I was too slow", "I reacted too quickly", or "I was faster than average in the computer exercise").

As a basic therapeutic rule, self-deprecation should be positively connoted according to the principle of reinforcement ("Those who work too quickly are prone to error"). Self-deprecating participants should also be reminded of possibilities for improvement ("Speed can be trained"). The functional relationship between pace and accuracy in the everyday lives of the participants thus becomes a key topic. The range of possibilities is marked by two extremes: "I'm fast but still free of error" and "I'm considered slow, and I also tend to make mistakes".

The results of the computer exercises, which have now been discussed, are then compared with previously recorded subjective performance assessments (▶ CD Worksheet 1). It should be taken into account that the computer-based results were obtained in laboratory-like conditions within the protected space of the therapy group. This performance thus cannot be compared directly with everyday performance, in which additional interactional and contextual demands are in play. For this reason, the next step is to read the first case vignette with the group.

▪ Case Vignette

One or more group participants read ▶ CD Vignette 1 paragraph by paragraph. After every section, the participants summarize the main ideas. The therapists direct their focus on the relationship between speed and alertness ("It was only because Peter was so alert that he could brake his bike in time"). After reading the case vignette, a group discussion is held with the following objectives:

- **Self-reference:** The participants identify themselves with particular aspects of the story ("The same thing happens to me") or distance themselves from them ("That's usually harder/easier for me").
- **Reference to everyday life:** Participants should identify and name concrete situations from their lives that they have experienced in a similar or contrary way to the case vignette's protagonist, Peter. At the end, the group should reach a common conclusion and find a title for the example situations. This can then serve as a guideline for subsequent discussion.

2.3.1.1.1.2 Attention/Vigilance

Attention/vigilance, the second neurocognitive target area of Module A, was already discussed in the introduction to the first target area, speed of information processing (e.g., "Those who work too quickly make more mistakes and vice versa"). To avoid thematic overlap, we first introduce the neurocognitive functional area of attention/vigilance. Then factors influencing speed of information processing and attention/vigilance are discussed as a group.

▪ Definition of the Target Area Attention/Vigilance

The neurocognitive function "attention" is defined briefly and in a generally understandable way. In the process, therapists should point out the distinction between attention activation (i.e., temporary power of concentration) and long-lasting maintenance of attention (vigilance):

Introduction Example

Attention is basically being able to concentrate on what is essential while having a conversation, working, or solving a task. Among other things, this requires that we hear and understand conversations, that we carry out activities at work, or that we perform tasks in a goal-directed way. For example: when we are having a conversation, we have to activate our attention as soon as someone speaks to us. If it is a longer conversation, we have to be able to hold our attention for a longer time.

To illustrate this, examples of deficits and resources are taken from everyday life:

- How many mistakes do I tend to make when I perform tasks?
- How exactly do I usually work or attend to things?
- How well can I concentrate on everyday tasks, e.g., reading a newspaper article or a letter, listening to a conversation, housekeeping, paying attention to traffic?

Therapists can also refer back to the experiences made with previously completed computer exercises.

? Key Question

- During the computer exercises, did I make more mistakes in the second half than in the first? (Refer to the feedback given by the program upon completion of a round of tasks)

▪ Promoting Self-Perception in the Cognitive Target Area

After this, participants take turns reporting on how they subjectively assess their own ability to concentrate and which situations they see their performance as weak or strong. Participants' statements regarding concrete situations are recorded on the flip chart. In addition, each participant fills out ► CD Worksheet 2 ("How well can I concentrate?"). The didactic approach is the same as that of the intervention unit on speed of information processing (see above). Also, therapists should point out the distinction between the short-term focusing of attention and longer-lasting power of concentration under low levels of stimulation.

▪ Case Vignette

The group now reads the case vignettes paragraph by paragraph (► CD Vignettes 2 and 3). In terms of content, these are a continuation of ► CD Vignette 1. ► CD Vignette 3 focuses on the theme of vocational rehabilitation. The protagonist Peter is confronted with the difficulty of having to maintain his power of concentration for a longer period of time.

After reading ► CD Vignette 2, a group discussion is held with the following goals:

- **Self-reference:** Participants identify themselves with particular aspects of the story ("The same thing happens to me") or distance themselves from them ("That's usually harder/easier for me").
- **Reference to everyday life:** The group compares the vignettes to situations from everyday life. Finally, a common conclusion and title for the example situations are found.

Only then is ► CD Vignette 3 read. This vignette introduces competitive work as a concrete target area when coping with difficulties in vigilance. Asking the participants about similar or contrary experiences reestablishes the connection to their everyday lives. In ► CD Vignette 3, factors affecting one's powers of vigilance (interest, states like boredom) are also addressed for the first time. The still highly structured group discussion is also centered on factors that influence one's power of concentration.

? Examples of Key Questions

- Is my power of concentration always the same?
- What does my ability to concentrate depend on?
- Can you give both a positive example of when you could concentrate well and a negative example? Can you describe these situations exactly?

Participants' everyday experiences concerning this cognitive target area are compiled on the flip chart and analyzed. The objective is a more discerning view of possible influences on attentional performance.

? Examples of Key Questions

- What was my mood in this situation?
- Did this activity interest and motivate me, or did it bore me?
- Did it demand too much or too little of me?
- Did I feel tired or awake?
- How was my daily rhythm at this time?

▪ Factors Influencing Performance in the Target Areas

While promoting self-reference and reference to everyday life as described above, participants often make the justified objection during group discussion that their cognitive performance in the target areas depends on numerous factors (e.g., mood, fatigue, medication). Thus, the next step is for the therapists to explore various influential factors that the participants experience in everyday activities. The aim is to establish an explicit connection between pace/attentional performance and the factors of alertness, daily rhythm, mood, medication, sleep, and lifestyle.

▪ The Influence of Alertness

With a view to INT's strict resource-orientation, the term "alertness" is used instead of "fatigue". For illustration, the alertness graph of a co-therapist or a participant – from waking in the morning to falling asleep at night – is shown on the flip chart as a model. This demonstrates the relationship between alertness and individual speed and attentional performance in the course of a day, Following this, each participant plots his or her average personal alertness graph on ► CD Worksheet 3 ("Alertness and speed/attention"). This should be confined to an average workday or the weekend. The worksheet can also be filled out as an independent exercise. However, this is only to be recommended for participants who are already highly motivated and active. The completed ► CD Worksheet 3 serves as a foundation for self-reference and reference to everyday life.

These questions are guidelines for the therapists for promoting participant self-reflection:

- When and where do I experience fatigue, sluggishness, and difficulty paying attention in my everyday life?
- When and where do I not?

In this way, the participant's subjective everyday experiences of personal strengths and weaknesses with respect to alertness, speed, and concentration are explored with the group and supplemented by ► CD Worksheet 3. In conclusion, performances in the target function, now felt as relevant to everyday experience, are compared with and contrasted to previous self-assessments of performance. In the process, the therapists stress the situation-specific resources of each participant and positively reinforce them. Finally, therapists draw attention to the cognitive performance profile of each participant – each characterized by individual strengths and weaknesses – according to the motto "Nobody is perfect!"

Now the topic of maintaining attention (concentration) over a long time period is discussed. Therapists should point out the differences between maintaining attention and speed of information processing or attention activation ("Before we wanted to be as alert and fast as possible during an activity. Now we are talking about keeping as alert as possible over a longer time period – at work for example – while making as few mistakes as possible"). Examples such as the following can be used for demonstration purposes:

In the Cockpit

A pilot is flying with his co-pilots and 100 passengers from Frankfurt over the Atlantic to New York. Flying time is 9 h. After starting, the pilots activate the autopilot, a kind of computer program for flying the airplane according to a preset route. We might think that the pilots have nothing more to do until landing in America. They could read a newspaper or sleep. There is also no variety during the trip. Flying high over the clouds, the pilots see almost nothing but white clouds and the blue sky above. There is no sensory stimulation. It is boring. Unfortunately, the pilots can't sleep, because they are responsible for over 100 passengers as well as the flight attendants. If something should happen (the airplane could experience wind turbulence, for example), the pilots have to react as quickly as possible and take control of the plane from the autopilot. In other words, they must always remain alert and capable of reacting very quickly, as we discussed on the topic of speed. They have to be able to maintain their alertness and attention from over 10 h, even when it is actually boring and nothing is happening. This is what we will talk about now.

In addition, the therapists can refer back to ► CD Vignettes 2 and 3 at this point. Again, the goal is to anchor the connection between alertness and sustained attention (vigilance) in the participants' everyday lives.

Examples of Key Questions

- In my everyday life, where does sustained attention play an important role? At work? In recreational activities? When I'm alone?
- Am I usually good at this?
- And do I feel alert and ready in the process?

The Influence of Medication

Patients often mention the negative side effects of neuroleptics as an influence on concentration and speed. Therapists should discuss patients' subjective experiences concerning such side effects on neurocognition in an approving and transparent way. To promote pharmacological compliance, patients should be reminded of the benefits of neuroleptic medication for coping with symptoms. They should also be reminded of positive experiences with new-generation neuroleptics. For this, easily comprehensible models and metaphors are best, such as are used in various psychoeducational approaches (see overview in Bäuml and Pitschel-Walz 2008). The island model created by Bäuml and his colleagues (Bäuml et al. 2010) for describing the dopamine hypothesis is provided here in an abbreviated form as an example:

Island Model for the Dopamine Hypothesis

Our brain contains a large amount of water. We can imagine the nerve cells in our brain as islands in an ocean that are in contact with each other. Thus, if we think or talk, the messages (information) are brought from one island to the next on boats (neurotransmitters, messengers). These boats land on different ports (receptors) on each island, and the cargo (message) is unloaded. The problem is that, if there is too much dopamine secretion under stress, too many boats are in transit, and the islands are overwhelmed with messages. The task of the neuroleptics is to block these island ports, reducing how many boats can land and thereby stopping the flood of messages. Older medications sometimes block too many ports, which with time gives us the feeling of being dulled. So newer medications purposely do not block all the ports. In this way, they assist communication, which we then experience as normal.

For illustration, a diagram of the island model is shown on the flip chart during the presentation.

If a patient's pharmacological noncompliance becomes a problem, the physician in charge should be contacted. The overriding goal is to point out the supportive effect of INT and comparable methods in re-attaining better cognitive performance. Psychotherapy – in conjunction with sociotherapeutic measures and medication – is a cornerstone of a successful multi-professional treatment.

The Influence of Interest and Motivation

The effect of interest and motivation on sustained attention is also an issue. In order to promote self-perception, the following resource-activating exercise can be carried out. A doctor's waiting room is simulated, complete with current newspapers and magazines on various subjects lying on the table. The participants should take a newspaper or magazine and browse through it. The aim is to activate the participants and to clarify the relationship between individual interests and attention.

Examples of Key Questions

- What attracts my attention?
- Where does my attention linger?

- What attracts my interest?
- What excites me?
- What motivates me? What excites me?

▪ The Influence of Mood

The topic of mood foreshadows the social-cognitive aspects of emotion perception as addressed in INT Module A (▶ Sect. 2.3.1.2). The therapists point out that mood or disposition affects attention. Moods themselves depend on the processing of internal and external stimuli. Not only our thoughts and feelings (including those directed towards the past or future) affect our mood; body perception does so too ("I feel sick/I have a headache"). By the same token, excessive or insufficient stimulation can lead to stress or apathy and boredom. To illustrate the connection between cognitive performance and mood, ▶ CD Information Sheet 2 ("Performance and mood") is distributed. The worksheet shows the influence of individual mood and the associated level of activation or excitement on (cognitive) performance. Highly chronic patients usually require extensive explanation of the activation graph.

The therapists call attention to the interaction between one's internal level of activation, feelings, or moods and cognitive performance. This INT intervention unit focuses initially on the lower (left) area of the activation graph on the worksheet, where the level of activation is too low to yield favorable cognitive-emotional coping. The goal is to explore states of mood that not only affect concentration negatively (during monotonous tasks in the workplace, for example) but can also detract from positive activities in leisure time. The first overriding topic is thus vigilance during understimulation. In almost every group constellation, there are participants who exhibit a generally high level of activation, who are anxious and distrustful, and who tend to become nervous when exposed to an overstimulating situation. Accordingly, these participants, due to increased distractibility, often experience attention and concentration problems even during activities that actually interest and motivate them. Should a participant have such an experience of increased activation and stress, this is acknowledged with the observation that the group will reflect more deeply on the topic of distractibility and overstimulation in the last part of INT (▶ Sect. 2.1). To avoid this situation, it is important that the patients can have positive experiences in this early phase of INT without much stress.

Recognizing the functional relationship between mood, activation, and cognitive performance is a key prerequisite for making a connection to the participant's everyday lives. The therapists again use the flip chart to record the everyday experiences discussed by the participants.

Finally, the focus is shifted to daily rhythm as another factor that affects attention. Daily rhythm depends on our individual lifestyle and how we structure our day. In this discussion, therapists can have recourse to the individual alertness graphs that each participant has already recorded on ▶ CD Worksheet 2. Attentional performance changes during the day are similar to those of alertness (e.g., "In the morning after waking I can't read a book, but I can in the evening"). When introducing this topic, therapists should also point out positive examples associated with experiences of success. For example, daily rhythm is determined to a great extent by quality of sleep (e.g., "When I don't sleep much, sometimes I hardly understand what people say to me" but "When I sleep well, sometimes I feel like I could take on anything"). A person's lifestyle manifests itself in his or her daily rhythm. Eating habits and the consumption of stimulants such as coffee, cigarettes, alcohol, and illegal drugs have an enduring effect on one's power of concentration. Participants' experiences in this regard are discussed and documented. Even if the consumption of alcohol and cannabis is not INT's primary focus of intervention, participants should be given time to discuss the issue if necessary so they can elaborate on the pros and cons of such consumption. The goal of this is reduction of consumption or abstinence. ▶ Chapter 3 includes tips on how to deal with patients for whom drug or alcohol abuse is a vital issue.

2.3.1.1.2 Compensation

The objective of compensation is to develop new coping strategies. The foundation for this is the concrete connection to patients' everyday lives and experiences that was made in the cognitive target area of speed of information processing. The next step is to individualize these strategies.

▪ Coping Strategies for Improving Speed and Attention Activation

On ▶ CD Worksheet 3, which was already used in the introductory sessions, the participants noted their own coping strategies for improving alertness, speed, and attention. (3rd question: "What can I change in order to be more alert, faster, and more attentive?"). These strategies are now neutrally compiled and recorded on the flip chart. Only then does the group discuss these suggestions and assess them for their own use in concrete situations.

? Examples of Key Questions

- Which strategy is promising and why?
- Which strategy improves my speed and attentional performance?
- Which strategies am I confident enough to try out in a certain situation?
- Which strategy suits me and which doesn't?

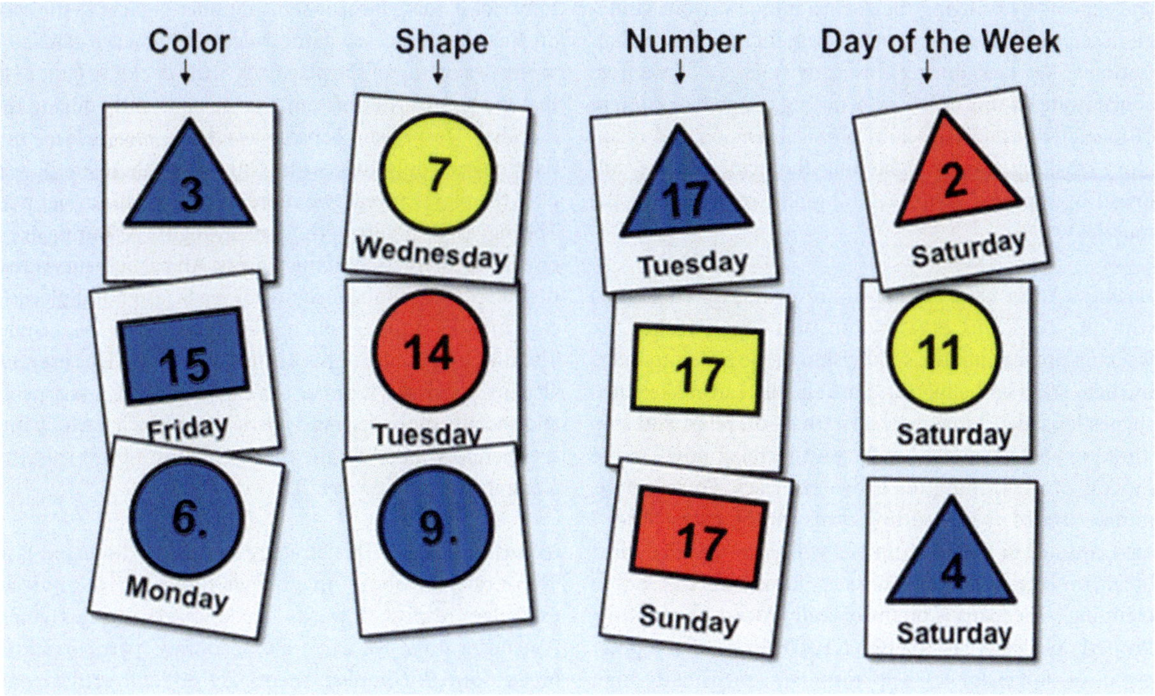

Fig. 2.3 IPT card-sorting exercise (Integrated Psychological Therapy, IPT, 1st Module; Roder et al. 1988, 2008a, 2010; with kind permission of Beltz Verlag)

Supplementing this, each participant receives ▶ CD Information Sheet 3 ("How do I have more speed and concentration"). This sheet lists strategies for the direct improvement of speed and preventative measures for indirect improvement. It also links speed with concentration, although the latter is discussed in the next intervention unit.

Repeated Practice This signifies the habituation of an activity until it becomes a routine. Simple exercises are carried out in the group for demonstration purposes. For example, one participant is asked to recite the alphabet or the numbers 1–50 as quickly as possible, while the other participants monitor how intelligible the letters or numbers are articulated and measure the time required. This exercise is repeated to demonstrate the effect of practice. The level of difficulty can be increased by saying the letters or numbers in reverse. Every round is followed by a feedback session. First the active participants are allowed to speak, then the observers, and finally the therapists. Another way to illustrate the effect of practice is by using the IPT card-sorting exercise (Roder et al. 1988, 2002, 2008a, 2010): each of the 230 cards has a design with four criteria: shape (round, triangular, or rectangular), color (blue, yellow, or red), number, and either no additional criterion or the name of a day of the week. None of the cards is identical to another. The enclosed ▶ CD-ROM includes examples of IPT cards (▶ CD Materials 1). The task is to sort the cards as quickly as possible according to a certain criterion, e.g., all cards with a blue design (▣ Fig. 2.3). When the time is stopped, other members of the group check to see whether mistakes have arisen during the sorting process. This exercise's level of difficulty can be varied by the number of cards or criteria to be sorted. In cases of low group cohesion or less capable participants, the exercise can be introduced briefly at the beginning before determining the target person. The participants are then asked how difficult the exercise is on a scale between 1 and 6, where 6 is the highest level of difficulty. Participants who assign it a low number are preferable for the exercise. As in all the following exercises, this exercise also concludes with a discussion of the strategy's everyday relevance.

Preventing Distraction In this context, this means directing one's attention to the task at hand (attention control) and repeatedly bringing the goal to mind. Various strategies are practiced in the group. These include self-verbalization ("My task during this activity is..."; "I want to concentrate on this task now"), noting the goal or content of the activity, and conscious physical tension and relaxation (making fists or tightening the arm muscles, followed by repeated deep breathing and relaxation of the muscles).

Having a Short Break Here we are primarily concerned with the conscious organization of a break within the working process and the subdivision of the task into intermediate steps and subgoals. Participants can make autosuggestions like "I may now take time out, relax, and stop thinking about the task" or "I want to relax now" in the process of performing the above exercises. For example, number series or IPT sorting cards can be used: "After I have counted or sorted 20 units, I will allow myself a short break, breathe deeply, and shake my arms before I proceed counting". The focus is on the overall process of counting. Properly placed breaks (between two rounds of computer exercises, for example) help sustain a consistently high speed of processing and ultimately lead more quickly to the final goal. The following section, "Coping strategies for maintaining attention/vigilance" contains a more detailed overview of the function of breaks in personally relevant domains such as work, recreation, and while reading.

Self-Motivation Following the principle of self-reinforcement, rewards for completed tasks are already planned beforehand: one may occupy oneself with something pleasant after the activity, treat oneself to something, or simply rest and do nothing. The aspect of self-determination – that we "may" do something, not "must" – is crucial. It can also help promote motivation if an activity is understood as a competition with oneself ("I want to be better than last time"). Light-hearted competition with others, as practiced in the following exercise, can also be motivating. The interaction-promoting card-sorting exercise "Speed" (▶ CD Materials 2a–l) consists of 96 cards each with different faces, colors, and numbers of faces. The faces express schematically depicted emotions, which can also be used as a preparation for the social-cognitive part of the module ("Which emotions are shown?"). In addition, there is one card with the game rules to be shown to the group (◘ Fig. 2.4). If the group is very large, it can be split in half and the exercise carried out simultaneously by both therapists in two smaller groups. In this case, the cards are printed out twice. Each participant receives one stack of concealed cards. One randomly selected card from the whole group is placed face-up in the middle. The aim is to place one's own cards on the play deck in the middle as quickly as possible according to certain criteria (either the same color, same face, or same number of faces as the card on the play deck; see game rules). Whichever card currently lies on top of the play deck is the deciding factor (so that the game criterion can change constantly during the exercise). To prevent sensory overload, every player initially reveals only two cards. Only when these are played does the player reveal two more cards from his or her pile. The biggest difficulty of this usually highly activating exercise is the interaction of the players. All participants reveal their cards simultaneously; whoever is faster and places a card first determines which playing card is in the middle. The first to place all of his or her cards wins. This exercise also involves risks: it can be too challenging for less capable and socially more reserved participants. Such participants are therefore aided by the therapists (prompting, playing along in teams of two, etc.).

Reducing Anxiety This strategy should be discussed last. The strategies above may seem indirectly to indicate excessive respect towards anxiety-inducing activities. Amending this, we can now encourage participants to break down a complex, seemingly difficult activity and always to begin with the easiest level of difficulty. In INT, this approach is followed particularly in the computer exercises. The error rate is reduced by this approach, providing more experiences of success and thus reducing anxiety. It should also be noted that paranoid-delusional distortions are not the focus of this intervention. Yet standardized cognitive restructuring is still possible: what causes the anxiety, which automatic assessments follow from this, and which alternative assessments are possible, each of which result in different consequences in thinking, feeling, and behavior? If this cannot be appropriately handled in the group because of excessive distrust, it can be discussed in additional one-on-one talks or be delegated to the therapist responsible for individual treatment.

Increasing Alertness by Motivation and Interest in the Activity to Be Completed The relationship between alertness and speed has already been discussed in detail. The target area of motivation and interest is introduced in the following intervention area. Therapists should therefore point out that a solution-oriented attitude often increases one's interest in the activity. The basis for this is the participants' insight into their own deficits and resources and related problems in the cognitive target area. Repeated emphasis of individual resources can be a particularly motivating factor in this process.

Sufficient Rest A balanced daily routine, based on a weekly structure and regular sleeping habits, can be a positive condition for speed in reasoning.

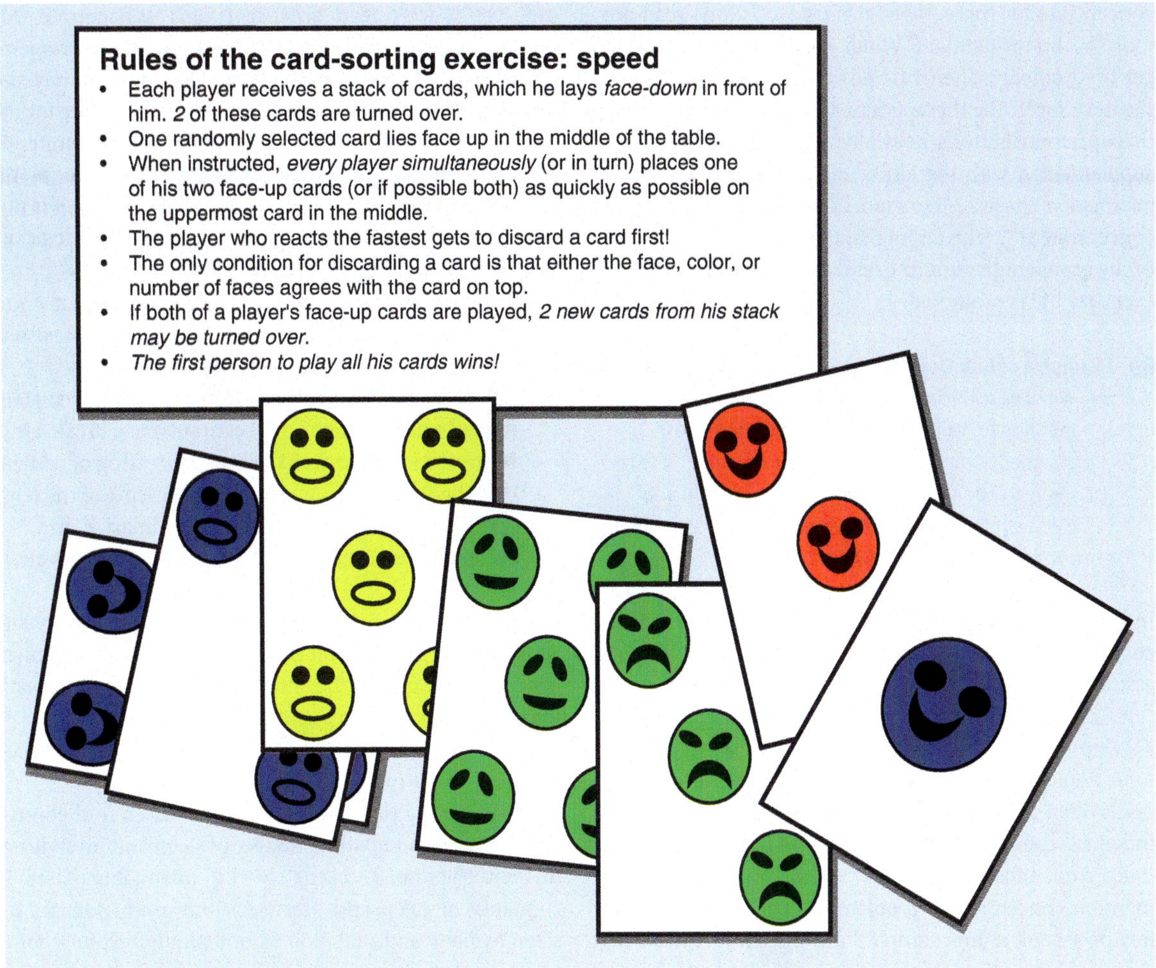

Fig. 2.4 Card-sorting exercise: "Speed"

If necessary, ► CD Information Sheet 3 can be supplemented with additional strategies. Finally, the coping strategies are individualized. Each participant assesses which strategies he or she would like to try out and which he or she does not feel confident about or considers unlikely to succeed. The aim of this intervention is to create an individual coping repertoire for each participant. These strategies are discussed again and again in the course of the treatment and are repeatedly applied, since speed is also related to other mental functions. As a result, there will continue to be a need to apply these coping strategies.

▪ Coping Strategies for Maintaining Attention/Vigilance

The overarching theme is the maintenance of attentional performance with little sensory stimulation. In contrast, the treatment focus of Module D is coping with stress caused by overstimulation. In the following section, individually applied strategies for maintaining attention – both successful and not so successful – are elicited and summarized on the flip chart. This is done with reference to everyday situations already recorded on the flip chart in the introductory section. Again, this procedure is resource-oriented.

? Examples of Key Questions

- In the situation described, what did I try to do to maintain my concentration?
- For what reasons and in which situations could I concentrate especially well? Can you tell us the trick you used to do it?

▪ Area-Specific Coping Strategies

The strategies can be subdivided into these basic rehabilitation domains: vocational ("Sometimes my work is boring. Then my thoughts drift and I need a break. After that my concentration is better again"), recreational ("I'm very motivated during longer activities that are meaningful to me, like sorting my extensive CD collection" or "Even when reading an interesting book, I could only concentrate for three pages at most, so I don't read anymore"), and residential ("When cleaning my apartment, I get tired quickly. Then I lie down and continue cleaning the next day"). The therapists first listen to and record participant contributions neutrally. These contributions are supplemented with the aid of the aforementioned ▶ CD Information Sheet 2 ("How do I become faster and more concentrated?"). The coping strategies are now discussed in the group, individualized, and a concrete connection to everyday life is promoted.

Examples of Key Questions

- We have summarized all the strategies we have mentioned for improving concentration and assigned some to the vocational domain, others to the recreational or residential domains. Which of these strategies do you think are promising for your own everyday life? Can you tell us why?

In the subsequent discussion, the therapists consciously encourage the use of arguments instead of assertions and assumptions.

Coping During Recreation

Incorporating the sphere of recreation supports a more discerning identification of resources and factors that influence concentration. These resources and factors can differ from those of the work sphere. Participants often mention concentration problems while reading a longer text or a book as an example from their free time. Using this problem point, the following will illustrate how to introduce new strategies for coping with concentration deficits and how to encourage practicing those strategies.

Concentration Problems While Reading

This intervention is optional and should only be introduced in the case of reading difficulties. First, the reading habits and needs of the participants are elaborated with a focus on resources.

Examples of Key Questions

- Do I like to read?
- What do I like to read?
- When and where do I like to read best?
- How much do I read in one sitting?
- What function does reading have for me? Or: Why don't I read?

Reading interests and functions can vary considerably. Individual experiences should be discussed (e.g., "I like to read detective novels", "I have to read textbooks for my education", or "I read to fall asleep"), including reasons for not reading (e.g., "I've never read a book. That's not for me", or "I don't read because I can't concentrate. My thoughts wander, and, at the end of a page, I can't remember what I just read"). Participants who claim to have no difficulties reading can act as a model and resource for the others. The group searches for possible reading strategies and both supplements and discusses these using ▶ CD Information Sheet 3 ("How do I have more speed and concentration?"). As a rule, group contributions can be assigned to three categories:

- **Prevent distraction:** self-verbalizations about attention control, reading out loud, taking notes on content, choosing an interesting text, etc.
- **Set subgoals and reduce self-expectations:** plan to read one chapter or one section, take a break, etc.
- **Memorize the content:** active processing of content (highlight or underline central statements of the text, take notes and write summaries, summarize the content in one's own words, repeat key passages etc.)

The group then practices the strategies it has found using short texts from periodicals or available books (implicit learning). The goal of this intervention is to improve reading ability and to reduce associated fears of failure.

Sleep Quality and Lifestyle

In the following step, ideas already discussed in the introductory section regarding quality of sleep and lifestyle are further elaborated. Using ▶ CD Information Sheet 4 ("Quality of sleep and lifestyle"), the group focuses on sleep hygiene and nutrition as potentially helpful coping strategies and risk factors for the power of concentration. The group reads the text section by section and discusses each point separately. The information sheet serves as an orientation aid. The initial goal of this intervention is to get the participants to look at their own life and sleeping habits critically and objectively. The next step is to promote appreciation of why an irregular daily routine and excessive consumption of stimulants are problematic. Finally, therapists encourage behavioral changes to reduce these risk factors. Participants can make concrete changes in their everyday lives in small steps in the form of independent exercises (see below: Independent Exercise). It is the responsibility of the therapists to prevent patients from having excessively high or stressful expectations of change (e.g., "I won't smoke any more starting tomorrow!"). These should be substituted with realistic goals (e.g., "Starting tomorrow, I'll try not to smoke before going to bed."). If individual goals concerning the topic areas discussed have already been introduced at this point (e.g., abstinence from or reduction of cigarette/alcohol consumption), these goals are noted and supported by the therapists. However, the focus here is on self-perception and willingness to change. The therapist may need to point out that they will concentrate on the concrete realization of individual goals in the "Problem Solving" section of Module C.

Coping Strategies During Work

A lot of rehabilitation effort is centered on the vocational domain, so work should be treated as a separate topic. Building upon the coping strategies already collected by the participants, various types of breaks and distraction strategies for increasing vigilance are introduced on ▶ CD Information Sheet 5 ("How can I concentrate better at work?"). The same group exercises are carried out, slightly modified, as in the previous intervention unit. However, they differ with respect to their aim: the focus is not on speed, but concentration (i.e., the number of errors). Again, implicit learning is stressed. This is achieved by involving active experiences and interactive practice. The following exercises are possible:

Reciting a Number Series or the Alphabet A participant is asked to recite the numbers 1 to 200 or the alphabet as correctly as possible, while the other participants monitor articulation and possible mistakes. Time is not measured. Instead, breaks, subgoals, self-verbalizations, and other previously mentioned strategies are deliberately applied. The level of difficulty can be increased by saying the letters or numbers in reverse. The round is immediately followed by a feedback session. First the active participants are allowed to speak, then the observers, and finally the therapists.

Card-Sorting Exercise This is a modification of the IPT card-sorting exercise (Roder et al. 1988, 2008a, 2010). Each participant receives 10–20 cards. Each card is characterized by four criteria: shape (round, triangular, or rectangular), color (blue, yellow, or red), number, and either no additional criterion or the name of a day of the week. Each participant now sorts his or her card pile according to a given criterion ("Please sort out all cards with a red shape"). Individualized strategies to improve concentration and reduce errors can be practiced again (e.g., self-verbalizations like "What is the task at hand? According to which criteria do I have to sort the cards?"). Each participant then monitors whether his or her neighbor has sorted the cards correctly. The level of difficulty of this exercise can be increased gradually by adding additional sorting criteria and more cards. However, the participants should have as successful an experience as possible so that the challenge boosts motivation, not stress.

Distraction Strategies The two exercises which have just been described are also used for trying out the distraction strategies contained on ▶ CD Information Sheet 5. In contrast to the speed exercises promoting attention activation, conscious and deliberate distraction now serves as a strategy for increasing attention when confronted with a monotonous activity with little sensory stimulation.

The experiences of the participants are compiled and their difficulties are analyzed. Therapists encourage the use of existing resources. The discussion should also address participants' particular work situations or employment programs.

Examples of Key Questions

- Did I use to take breaks consciously during work?
- How often and how long did I require breaks to be so I could recoup and concentrate better?
- Which distraction strategies for improving concentration would I like to try out during work?
- What difficulties do I expect?

Card-Sorting Exercise for Mood and Concentration

At the end of the compensation section of this intervention unit, direct reference is made to the social-cognitive components of Module A (▶ Sect. 2.3.1.2) by linking concentration and mood. This also reintroduces the topics of alertness and speed/attention (▶ CD Worksheet 3), cognitive performance and mood (▶ CD Information Sheet 2), and related participant experiences. The group now performs the card-sorting exercise "Mood and Concentration". A total of 29 cards are found on the enclosed ▶ CD-ROM (▶ CD Materials 3a and 3b). On the 27 smaller cards are concepts concerning emotional states. On the two large cards are printed the two polar opposites "Alert and Concentrated" and "Tired and Distracted". These latter two cards are either attached to the flip chart or are each assigned to one of the two therapists. In the latter case, one therapist is considered alert, the other tired. The cards indicating emotional states are distributed among the participants. The participants now take turns assigning the cards to one of the alertness poles. The currently active participant should also justify his or her assignment with an argument based on everyday experiences. Cards for which no consensus is found in the ensuing group discussion and cannot be assigned unambiguously to one of the alertness poles are placed between the two large cards. The point of the exercise is not group consensus but to encourage the formation of understandable arguments based on patients' own experiences (◘ Fig. 2.5).

To make more use of group dynamics, the exercise can alternatively be carried out by splitting the group into two halves. One half of the group gets the "Alert and Concentrated" card, the other the "Tired and Distracted"

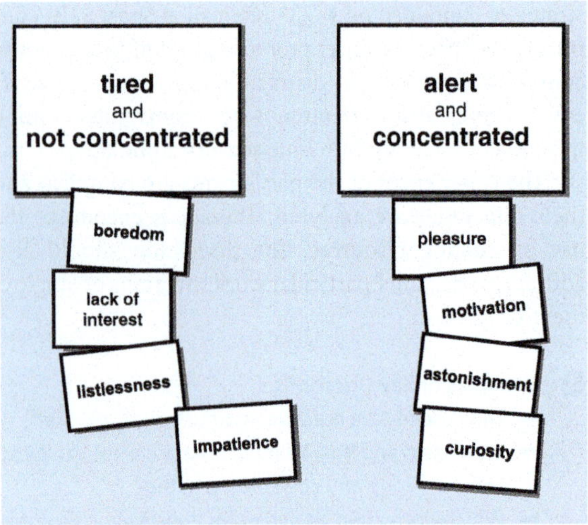

Fig. 2.5 Card-sorting exercise: mood and concentration

card. To assist the participants in their assessment of the cards, the therapists begin by updating the connection between the two poles of alertness and the internal activation level (excitement, arousal) with the help of ▶ CD Worksheet 2 and ▶ CD Information Sheet 3. The two groups then determine which activation level corresponds to their pole of alertness. The cards are sorted and distributed randomly. The task of both groups is to discuss which cards do not belong to their activation level and to exchange them with the other group. If the entire group is in agreement, the emotions are read aloud. The group then discusses whether the assignment seems realistic. The aim of this exercise is that the participants assign equivalent internal activation levels to different emotions. In this phase of INT, patient self-reference remains limited to motivational feeling states that tend to accompany understimulation, such as boredom, loss of motivation, listlessness, disinterest, apathy, dejection, lack of energy. In order to promote self-perception of such moods and willingness to change, it is important to emphasize positive moods. The participants should learn that increased internal excitation (arousal) and concentration need not only be associated with negative emotions, but is also linked to positive feeling states like hope, interest, joy, challenge, motivation etc.

If the group already has a high level of cohesion and contains motivated, resourceful participants, the following variation is possible: the emotional states written on the cards can initially be represented nonverbally by one participant or two participants simultaneously. The other group members cannot see the term being depicted. Then the group determines the level of activation being expressed and tries to assign the feeling that has been shown to tiredness or alertness. A distinction is made in the process between the levels of description, perception, and interpretation.

Examples of Key Questions
- Which facial expressions, gestures, and behavior patterns are being shown?
- When I see such behavior patterns, which expressions of emotion do I generally perceive?
- When I or others feel such an emotion, do I tend to feel excited (high activation) or not?
- Is this expression of emotion (and the associated level of activation) related more to tiredness or to alertness?

Summing up, this exercise pursues two goals:
1. Sensitizing the participants to the distinction between subjectively experienced emotions and objective, visible observations of associated behavior and linking these emotions to concentration, and
2. Preparing participants for the social-cognitive content of Module A (▶ Sect. 2.3.1.2), emotion perception.

2.3.1.1.3 Restitution

Repeated Practice in the Area of Speed of Information Processing

In this target area, the restitution section comprises above all the repetition of computer-based exercises, which have already been worked on briefly in the introductory sessions. The card-sorting exercises (▶ CD Materials 1, 2a–l) described above can also be repeated to create a more relaxed atmosphere. The restitution section serves to rehearse the coping strategies developed in the compensation section to the point of habituation. When preparing an exercise, each participant should fill out ▶ CD Worksheet 4 ("My helpful strategies for …") individually.

Computer-Based Exercises

The method always follows the principles of "errorless learning": participants begin with the exercise level that is simplest for them in order to keep the amount of errors low and maximize their experience of success. Only when the participant has mastered this basic level does he or she proceed to the next level. At least 80 % of the tasks within an exercise should be solved correctly to be successful. In the following speed exercises, it is sometimes impossible to measure performance. In such cases, performance should be assessed by a therapist. Because the tasks are done individually, both the pace and the number of processed tasks vary among the participants. After some have finished all the available tasks, others have not come any further than the first two levels of difficulty. For this reason, therapists should positively reinforce slower participants constantly. If necessary, they should be given temporary individual assistance in working out the tasks. Before the participants begin working at their computers, the primary therapist demonstrates the exercise at his or her computer while a digital projector displays the image on a screen. The trial run contained in every CogPack exercise lends itself to this. Therapists should select exercises that are relevant on the problems under focus. Both the severity of the participants' cognitive impairments and their resources should determine the difficulty level of the exercises and how many should be undertaken. The following CogPack exercises have proven effective:

VISUMOTOR It is recommended that therapists start with this CogPack exercise, as it is especially suitable for introducing the group to the program. The first two sub-exercises are relatively easy to master. This helps to reduce anxiety and gives the participants a feeling of success. The easiest exercise is exercise a (Follow the Road). Following this, exercises b (Steer the Raft, easy) and c (Steer the Raft, hard) should be done. Because of their higher level of difficulty, exercises d and e (Follow a Target slow/fast) are optional and recommended only for especially capable participants.

UFOs This classic reaction speed exercise is highly stimulating because of the moving stimuli and game-like approach. The following tasks are recommended: a (slow large UFOs), b (small fast UFOs), and c (hypers). The level of difficulty increases from a to c. Task d (ultras) is not appropriate since performing this task correctly can be very difficult depending on the display quality. In e (permanently adaptive UFOs), the program adjusts the difficulty level to the previous performance of the participant.

FALLINGSTARS This exercise has a structure similar to the UFO exercise above. The level of difficulty increases gradually from a (easy) to b (intermediate) to c (hard). The "hard" exercise requires some practice to master. In d (adaptive), the program adjusts the difficulty level to the previous performance of the participant.

BALL As an alternative to UFO, the equally activating BALL exercises can be utilized. The level of difficulty increases from task a to task f, and exercises with or without sound can be selected.

STOP Here, the user must click on a clock at a given time. There are three levels of difficulty. An analog clock (a-c) or a digital clock (d-f) can be selected.

REACTION Five reaction exercises are recommended (a-e). In these, the reaction time for correct clicking is measured in addition to the number of errors. This task helps clarify the connection between speed and number of errors.

Usually, not all of the exercises listed above are carried out. After a maximum of 30 min, the group returns to the group room. The group then discusses their experiences with the exercises in a feedback session. In this session, therapists direct the group's attention to the coping strategies that were involved. Difficulties and successful experiences that arose in the course of repeated practice are also addressed.

Examples of Key Questions
- What strategies did I employ? Which were helpful and which not? Could I apply the strategies immediately or did I need repeated practice?
- How did I experience the exercises? Did I improve with time or not? What is the reason for this?
- Did I profit sufficiently from repeated practice or do I need more practice?

The therapists have actively accompanied the individual exercises and have already given feedback (as positive as possible) on performance. They now structure the discussion in such a way that the participants assess their own performance as adequately as possible. For this purpose, therapists can remind the group of the self-assessments they made about speed of information processing, using ▶ CD Worksheet 1 as a reference.

Examples of Key Questions
- Did my speed improve during the last few sessions?
- Do I assess my speed exactly the same now as I did when we began this topic?

Each participant makes a note of any changes on ▶ CD Worksheet 1 and corrects previous self-assessments if necessary.

Repeated Practice in the Area of Maintaining Attention/Vigilance

The restitution section on vigilance is divided between the repetition of CogPack exercises in the computer room and the aforementioned card-sorting exercises in the group therapy room. The aim is to practice to the point of habituation strategies offered by participants and those on ▶ CD Information Sheets 2–5 and ▶ CD Worksheet 3 for improving vigilance.

Card-Sorting Exercises

The card-sorting exercises described above (▶ CD Materials 1, 3a–b) are now repeated. The following is a possible variation of the IPT card-sorting exercise (▶ CD Materials

1) (described in Roder et al. 2010): every participant and both therapists receive 6–8 IPT cards each (▶ CD Materials 1) which they spread face up on the table. The co-therapist or one of the participants now has the task of selecting one of the displayed cards. With a group size of eight participants and two therapists, 60 or 80 cards are used. The co-therapist or selected participant notes the card's features on a sheet of paper in such a way that the other players cannot see it. The task of the rest of the group is to find out what the target card is by asking specific questions about its features. The participant who selected the cards may only answer with "yes" or "no". Most groups soon think of turning over cards that have been ruled out to reduce the card selection. The exercise's difficulty level can be increased if the group has to avoid "no" answers or they must first determine which person is sitting in front of the target card.

▪ **Computer-Based Exercises**

The CogPack program contains various vigilance exercises. The following have proved effective in INT:

PIECE-WORK Various sorting tasks simulate the kind of sensory understimulation that is characteristic of work on an assembly line. The amount of understimulation can be varied by changing the speed of the conveyor belt. This option can help promote self-perception in the following way: 1. each participant selects the speed they are most comfortable with, and 2. the speed that causes the most discomfort. The participant then practices under both conditions. Exercises (a-d) (high/low fences and large/small blocks) differ only with respect to the stimuli presented, not in terms of the level of difficulty. Exercise e (tiles) contains model blocks that are difficult to distinguish. Accordingly, this exercise is only used towards the end of the intervention.

SEQUENCE This exercise is similar in structure to the Continuous Performance Test (MATRICS Assessment, Inc. 2006). Feedback is given only after the exercise is completed. A total of 19 SEQUENCE exercises of about 3 min duration are available. Exercise a "numbers" is recommended to start with, since it requires the lowest skill level. Besides this, these exercises have also proved effective: b and c (numbers), d (alphabet), and e-h with sequences of days of the week, months, seasons, and dates. In addition, exercise i (traffic lights) contain figural stimuli.

SCAN These exercises differ from the two mentioned above. Here, the duration of the exercise depends on the working pace of the participants. The time needed for completion is measured. Errors are penalized with penalty seconds. The host of stimuli that must be processed tests the participants' power of vigilance. Tasks a-h differ with respect to the target stimuli.

In working out these exercises, participants habituate the coping strategies that were individualized in the compensation section. Self-perception is also promoted. The direct feedback given by CogPack after each exercise sequence is an initial didactic means to this end: was there an increase or a decrease in performance from the first to the second half of the exercise sequence?

After a computer exercise session, generally 30 min long, participants engage in self-perception by reflecting on individual experiences in the group room.

? Examples of Key Questions
- Did I find the exercise easy or difficult?
- Was the exercise monotonous and boring?
- Did I become fatigued and increasingly less concentrated during the exercise?

Therapists then recall the factors influencing concentration discussed in the compensation section of this module.

? Examples of Key Questions
- What made the exercises boring?
- When were they interesting?
- Why was I (not) interested, motivated, enthusiastic?
- How was my mood during the exercises?

Finally, experiences with practiced coping strategies are discussed.

? Examples of Key Questions
- Could I concentrate on the task until the end?
- What helped me do this? What did I try out?
- Were the strategies we discussed helpful? Did they give me additional stress or perhaps motivate me?

Group discussions of the exercises are also always focused on resources. Participants' strengths are stressed more than their deficits. Especially the PIECE-WORK exercises, with a duration of 15 min, is borderline over-demanding for some participants. It is important for such participants to have the option of not working through the exercise to the end. Instead, the shorter SCAN or SEQUENCE exercises can be done. The difficulties of some participants may be attributable to impairments of selective attention in conjunction with the experience of stress. If so, Module

D should be consulted. Finally, each participant should amends his or her current self-assessment of concentration on ▶ CD Worksheet 2.

2.3.1.1.4 In Vivo Exercises and Independent Exercises

One important goal the in this first intervention unit of Module A has been boosting participants' motivation to participate actively and to promote group cohesion. For this reason, carrying out in vivo and independent exercises at this stage of the INT process is considered optional. Participants should consider which of the strategies and experiences discussed in the group they can also use in their own everyday lives. To aid this process, each member of the group fills out ▶ CD Worksheet 5 (independent exercise). Therapists describe the topic of the independent exercise and introduce the concrete situation to be expected. They also suggest the strategy to be employed. Feared or expected difficulties are also anticipated. After experiencing the target situation concretely, the participants can note any difficulties that arose. If independent exercises are assigned, they should be discussed in the following session. Difficulties and are addressed as well as successes. If group cohesion is already high, the group should also motivate participants who initially refused to do independent exercises at the next opportunity. However, the intensity and frequency of independent exercises should always be adapted to group composition and participant motivation and performance.

As supplements or alternatives to independent exercises, in vivo exercises are provided. In these, the participant tries to apply new coping strategies for improving speed or attention/vigilance in a real, on site situation. However, this intervention depends on the composition of the group, on local conditions, and not the least on the time resources of the therapists and participants. In vivo exercises demand considerable time in preparation, execution, and subsequent discussion. For example, if there are facilities for occupational therapy in the immediate vicinity, the group can accompany the participant concerned into his or her protected workplace. There the participant can apply coping strategies on site and observing participants can learn by example. In vivo exercises are also possible in the recreational and residential spheres. The group can go on a short excursion, for instance. Before any of these joint activities, the patients involved should fill out ▶ CD Worksheet 4 ("My helpful strategies for…"). This helps the participant become more focused on the approaching task. Each in vivo exercise concludes with a debriefing session.

2.3.1.2 Social-Cognitive Intervention Area: Emotion Perception

Module A: Social-Cognitive Intervention Area: Emotion Perception

1. Introduction
   - Definition: emotion perception
   - Self-perception in the target area
   - Filter model
   - Resource-oriented individual profile in the target area
   - Connection to self and everyday life: case vignette
   - Definition and functions of basic emotions
2. Compensation
   - Learning coping strategies for emotion-decoding in 3 stages: facial perception, facial expressions and gestures, emotion sequences
   - Personal expression of emotion in group exercises
   - Emotional concept formation
3. Restitution
   - Habituation of learned coping strategies in repeated group exercises
4. In vivo exercises and independent exercises
   - Transfer of individualized coping strategies to concrete, everyday situations

Tips

- Infrastructure: group therapy room, flip chart, projector
- Therapy materials: ▶ CD Information Sheets 6–8, ▶ CD Worksheets 4–5, ▶ CD Vignette 4, Ekman pictures (▶ CD Materials 4a–b), ▶ CD e-Materials 1–3; card-sorting exercise: emotional concepts (▶ CD Materials 5a–h)
- Didactics: highly structured group discussion

2.3.1.2.1 Introductory Sessions

▪ Definition of the Target Area

The social-cognitive function of emotion perception has already been introduced in the neurocognitive intervention section of Module A. This intervention concerned the effect of mood on neurocognitive functioning. The present topic is recognizing the feelings and emotional states of other persons. First the concept of emotion perception should be defined.

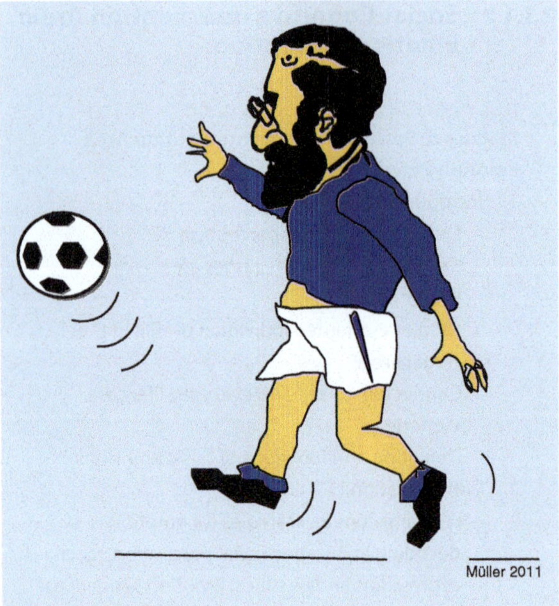

Fig. 2.6 "Love or football, that is the question!"

Introduction Example

Our thoughts, actions, and bodily sensations are related to our feelings. For example, when we laugh, cry, or swear, we express our feelings in a way that is easy for others to recognize. It's difficult not to express feelings. Every feeling or emotion we experience is characterized by certain modes of expression such as facial expressions, gestures, and behavior. These can be identified by others.

Therapists also point out the value of the skill of correctly perceiving the emotions of others.

Introduction Example

Being able to assess the emotions expressed in a conversation or in public provides a sense of security and helps in orientation. A person's emotional expression can often be recognized even when that person says nothing or the other does not hear what is being said (nonverbal behavior). A gesture or facial expression is often worth a thousand words. From emotions, we recognize what attitude a person has towards another: Does the person have a positive or negative attitude? Does the person bear a grudge or is he/she friendly? On the other hand, a false interpretation of emotions often leads to uncertainty, fear, or to groundless distrust.

▪ Optical Illusions (Optional)

As an option, optical illusions or tilted images can be used to introduce perception processes in a relaxed atmosphere. Numerous books and Internet sites contain an extensive amount of illustrations, which can be used by therapists. Figure 2.6 is one example of such an illustration.

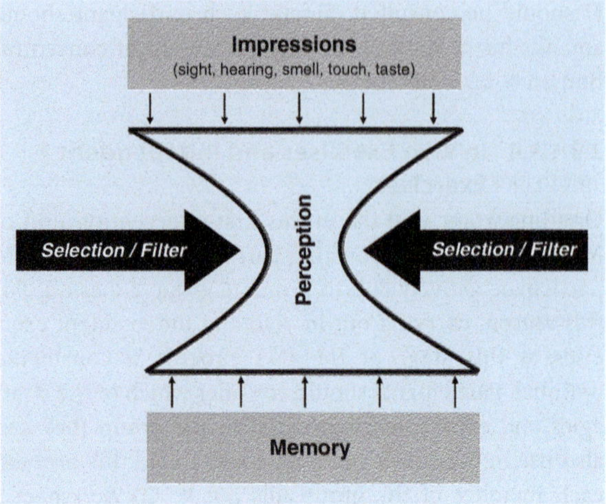

Fig. 2.7 Filter model: perception and memory (Müller and Roder 2012)

▪ Filter Model

One overriding didactic goal throughout the INT process is to make connections between the various intervention units as they follow in succession. A newly introduced intervention area thus always refers to directly preceding units. This promotes intrinsic motivation. Participants can understand why it is important to spend time (just now) on this intervention area.

Here, we review previously discussed factors influencing speed and attentional performance such as one's current mood and emotional state. This is done in the light of a participant's own experience and those of his or her intervention partners. For this purpose, the filter model of perception is introduced. This is available both for electronic presentation (▶ CD e-Materials 1) and as an information sheet (▶ CD Information Sheet 6) since it will be used again and again in subsequent intervention units (Fig. 2.7).

The filter model is used to illustrate basal perception processes. Perception with the five senses is discussed, and then the connection between perception and memory (an intervention of Module B) is established. Finally, therapists talk about various filters that affect information selection (selective perception is an intervention area of Module D). If filters shaped by attitude and personality are mentioned in the process, the participant is referred to the social-cognitive section of Module C. Using participants' everyday examples, therapists relate the topic back to that of attention and interest as well as the level of alertness. The everyday examples of the group help to individualize the significance of emotions for perception and memory and to exemplify the filter modalities. Yet the primary topic is the effect of personally experienced emotions on perception. It is recommended that this subject matter be illustrated with simple examples:

Filtering Perception
A participant is asked whether she has already seen the person sitting next to her and has spoken to that person. This participant answers in the affirmative. The person is asked to maintain eye contact with the therapist who is speaking and not to look at the neighbor. The next question is whether the participant can describe in detail the shoes her neighbor is wearing.

Emotional Influences on Perception
A participant is asked whether he likes pizza. In case he says yes, the therapist asks what his favorite pizza is. The therapist then asks whether the participant can imagine the following: he is walking home this evening with a growling stomach. As he passes by a pizzeria, he can smell the wonderful aroma of pizza baking in real wood-fired oven. He yields to the aroma, goes in, and orders his favorite pizza. If the participant can imagine this, the therapist then asks about the emotions he might experience in such a situation. The scenario continues: unfortunately, one of the pizza ingredients was no longer fresh, and he winds up having to spend most of the night on the toilet. Finally, he walks past the pizzeria 1 week later (after the group session), again smelling the aroma of pizza from the wood-fired oven. The final question is then: "Did the smell of the pizza trigger the same emotions as it did last week?"

▪ Promoting Self-Perception in the Cognitive Target Area

The group first focuses on recognizing the emotional expressions of others in social interaction. Within the structure of INT, this serves as the prerequisite for the social-cognitive functions, discussed later in Module B, of ToM and social perception. These functions build upon proficiency in adequate affect decoding. The therapists could introduce the subject in the following manner:

Introduction Example
We have dealt with the significance of emotions for perception and concentration. In social situations, when we meet other people, emotions are also being expressed constantly – emotions which we can perceive and recognize. Recognizing the emotions of others makes it possible for us to orient ourselves very quickly regarding how the other person is doing and how that person feels about us. The emotional involvement of our conversation partners and our own emotional involvement help us to recall these situations and experiences.

By linking affective activation with the power of memory, we have anticipated the intervention area of Module B (verbal and visual memory). The point here is to bring into focus participants' self-perception of their ability to perceive emotion.

Participants are each asked how they assess their own ability to recognize emotions expressed by other people.

? Examples of Key Questions
- Do you consider it easy or difficult to recognize emotions expressed by others and to interpret them correctly?
- In which concrete situations and under what conditions is it easier to do this?
- What are the pros and cons of being immediately able to identify emotions?
- When another person expresses an emotion, does this lead to uncertainties?

In addition, each participant fills out ► CD Worksheet 6 ("How well can I recognize the feelings of others?"), which is discussed according to the method described above.

▪ Case Vignette

Participants take turns reading ► CD Vignette 5 paragraph by paragraph. In this short story, the protagonist Peter has a date with Manuela, a woman he likes. This story indirectly introduces the target area and demonstrates INT's didactic questioning technique.

Discussion of Content First the group summarizes and discusses the story section by section to promote understanding of its content. Also, therapists activate the participants by asking how they assess the chances for another encounter with Manuela (open-ended story).

Promoting Argumentation Therapists encourage the formulation of arguments based on facts (e.g., Peter has good chances because Manuela came early to the meeting place and said goodbye with a warm handshake). Assertions and assumptions are scrutinized with the help of existing facts (cognitive conversation techniques; Socratic dialog).

Definition of the Target Area The emotion expressed by Manuela in the story is discussed as a potential argumentation aid ("How do I recognize in Manuela's face whether she is expressing pleasure, annoyance, or disgust?")

Self-Reference The participants are asked about their own experiences and how they deal with perceiving emotions. Positive and negative experiences are compared and possible influential factors are analyzed ("Are there situations and condition under which I succeed better in assessing emotions than in others? What does this depend on?").

Reference to Everyday Life The concern here is to sensitize patients to the relevance of the target area to coping with everyday life. Concretely experienced situations from individual everyday experience are described in detail.

Again, the flip chart is used to compile contributions to the discussion. Therapists should take care that the discussion is not limited to facial expressions and gestures, which are often mentioned first; the entire palette of human modes of expression emotions should be taken into consideration. If concrete emotions are mentioned, these can also be shown and expressed by the therapists and patients. However, expressing emotional states via facial expression and gestures or by modifying speech volume can be a potential stress factor for some participants. If there is a danger of this, therapists should structure the discussion to avoid this. The co-therapist or a participant with suitable resources can be used as a model. Participants with greater deficits (those with pronounced negative symptoms with increased flattening of emotions, for example) should always be supported in a playful group atmosphere and should be positively reinforced when they present something.

Definition of Basic Emotions

The aim of this intervention is to differentiate the concept of emotion, which has hitherto been treated non-specifically, and finally to categorize it. Together, the group defines basic, culturally independent emotions.

Examples of Key Questions

- What basic emotions are expressed and experienced more or less the same in all cultures?
- What effect do these emotions have on me?
- Do I perceive them as pleasant or not?
- How do I usually deal with them?

All emotions discussed in the group are collected and compiled on the flip chart. As a rule, a large number of emotion concepts can be complied in this way, far surpassing the amount of basic emotions defined in the literature. It is thus up to the therapists to lead the subsequent discussion with focused questioning such that these concepts are assigned to categories (e.g., the concept "fun" can be assigned to the general term "pleasure", "disgruntled" to the general concept "anger", "amazement" to "surprise", or "depressed" to "grief"). These categories correspond to the basic emotions. The conceptualization of emotions described here will again be the subject of a card-sorting exercise in the following compensation section. The following basic emotions are target areas in the associated INT module "Emotion Recognition":

- pleasure
- anger/rage
- anxiety/fear
- disgust
- grief
- surprise

The therapists also confirm other emotions such as shame or love, but they are not handled in the following compensation exercises (stage 1). In the first phase of this intervention unit, the stress level of the participants should be kept as low as possible. Feelings of shame and, for many participants, of love are often associated with unpleasant, stressful experiences. States of emotion are discussed, but stresses linked to them will be the subject of interventions in Module D (emotion regulation). The same is true of participants' subjective experience of negative emotions like sadness or highly activating feelings like fear, rage, and anger. It should also be taken into account that even emotions that are positive per se like happiness can be perceived in a stressful way by the patients ("I can't be happy anymore", "I have a bad conscience when I'm happy"). Also, the basic emotion of surprise can have both positive and negative components ("It's a pleasant surprise when someone invites me to a coffee" vs. "I don't like to be surprised with an invitation to a drink. Then I don't know what the other person wants from me in return").

Function of Emotions

Some participants may comment that emotions are pointless because they often involve stress or pressure and are themselves perceived as such. Thus, it is necessary to focus also on the function of emotions. The ultimate purpose is to promote the recognition of emotions and, later in Module D, the regulation of emotions. Here are some possible guidelines:

- **Every emotion always has a certain function:** When we experience a feeling ourselves or perceive the emotions of others, we obtain important information this way. Emotions are carriers of useful information.
- **Pleasure:** Pleasure gives us a feeling of happiness. People like to communicate pleasure, and this can be contagious.
- **Anger:** When we aren't satisfied with ourselves, feel provoked by our environment, we signal this by showing anger. Everyone then immediately recognizes that something doesn't suit us, and at the moment it's best not to tangle with us. Anger and rage are also valves for releasing pressure.
- **Fear:** This feeling warns us about danger and reminds us to be careful. Something that might happen may or may not be predictable (e.g., "A deer relies on its fear so that it will be careful and avoid becoming the prey of predators or hunters.")
- **Disgust:** Like fear, disgust can also warn us of danger. Disgust warns us not to come too close to

certain things or not to eat what might be bad for us. Disgust is directed towards particular, concrete objects. It is caused by smell, taste, contact, or appearance.

- **Grief:** With this we express the loss of a person close to us, not only when someone dies, but also when someone leaves us. Grief usually lasts a long time and helps us to process our longing for the lost person and our pain. We can also react with grief when we have not reached a goal. This feeling is shorter in duration, however.
- **Surprise:** This feeling is a direct reaction to something unexpected that does not correspond to our experience. This can be experienced positively or negatively. If we are surprised, we are initially in shock before we attempt in our astonishment to classify the situation and react to it. With surprise, we signal that we did not expect what has happened and that our reaction to it will be spontaneous.

The discussion now centers on the relevance of these emotions to the everyday lives of the participants. Everyday experiences of each basic emotion are compiled in the group. The group also discusses how high their level of activation (internal excitation) was in these situations along with their degree of alertness and the emotion's effects on concentration. Deciding what is "right" or "wrong" is not the focus. Instead, the aim is to promote the self-perception of emotions experienced in everyday life.

2.3.1.2.2 Compensation

In the compensation section, the group now works out techniques for recognizing emotions by means of facial expressions. In addition to facial expressions, gestures are also addressed as possible ways to express emotions. Finally, the group's attention will be turned to sequences of emotion often experienced and observed in everyday life. Emotion decoding is split into three stages:

1. affect decoding using facial perception,
2. affect decoding using facial expressions and gestures, and
3. emotional sequences.

A variety of pictorially represented stimuli exists for this purpose. This material is available in electronic form for presentation with a projector (▶ CD e-Materials) or, for stage 1, should be acquired on the Internet. The goal of the compensation section is that each participant becomes acquainted with compensation strategies. Participants then practice applying the new affect-decoding techniques in the group context. Compensation then concludes with a card-sorting exercise on emotional concept formation, in which further emotions and other ways to express basic emotions are clarified.

▪ Affect Decoding Stage 1: Facial Perception

Stage 1 focuses on the perception of the face when recognizing emotions. For illustration, individual images of facial expressions on the accompanying ▶ CD-ROM can be utilized (▶ CD Materials 4a–b; pictures with emotions; stage 1).

? Examples of Key Questions

- From what facial features can we recognize a feeling being expressed?
- How do the basic emotions we discussed differ with respect to these features? For example, how does fear differ from pleasure or grief?

The contributions are collected and supplemented with the tips on ▶ CD Information Sheet 7 ("How do I recognize the feelings of others?"). The group discusses various features of facial expressions for each of the six basic emotions: shape and position of the eyes, eyebrows, eyelids, nose, and mouth; lines in the corners of the mouth, on the nose, between the eyebrows, and on the forehead. The emotionally neutral face is also introduced as a reference point for differentiating expressions of emotion (▶ CD Information Sheet 7). Each participant should be able to recognize and distinguish the basic emotions with the help of various features of facial expression.

Affect decoding techniques that have been learned are now practiced for the first time in the group. The pictures contained on the enclosed ▶ CD-ROM are especially suitable for this. Each picture shows a face expressing a basic emotion (▶ CD Materials 4a–b; affect decoding stage 1; facial expressions). These frequently used pictures by Ekman and Friesen (1976) have been standardized. Only those pictures are included that were assigned to one of the basic emotions in a standardization population with at least 70 % agreement. There is a total of 82 pictures (◘ Fig. 2.8). These are subdivided into pictures with faces expressing either fear, anger, disgust, pleasure, grief, or surprise. Emotionally neutral faces are also depicted as control stimuli.

The purpose of this compensation section is for participants to apply emotion recognition techniques for the first time and to promote self-perception of skills in this cognitive functional area. In the restitution section following this, newly learned techniques are habituated via repeated practice. For this reason, initially only 1–2 pictures are used for each basic emotion. The pictures are presented with the projector. The group should identify the basic emotion being displayed using objectively identifiable features of facial expressions. Again, the goal is to compile objective facts of feeling perception and to separate speculations and hypotheses. Finally, the pictures of basic emo-

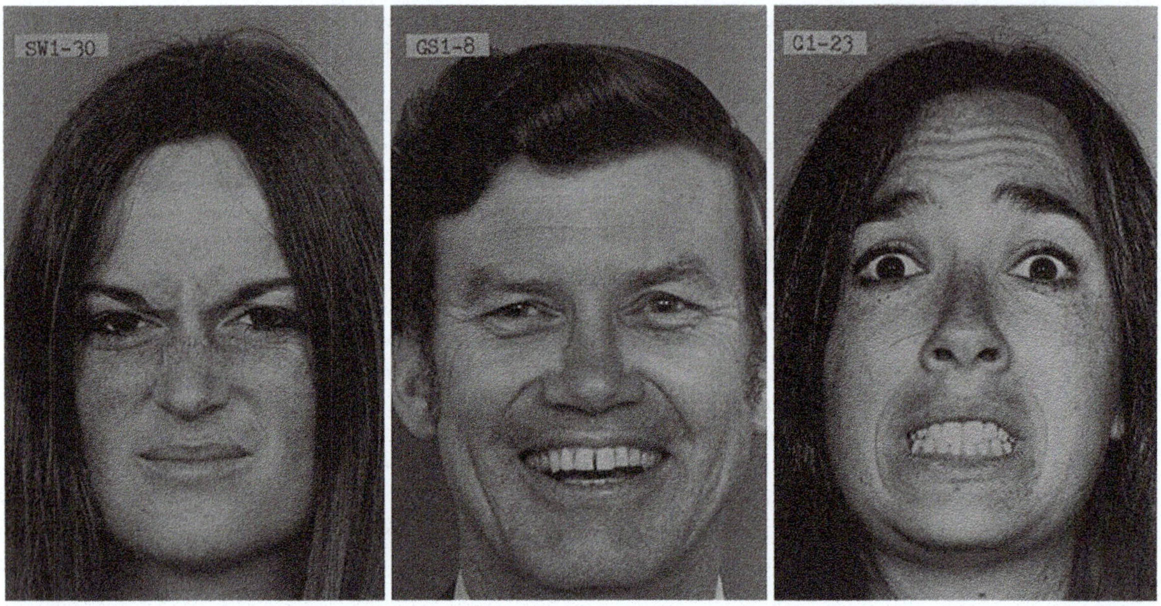

Fig. 2.8 Affect decoding stage 1: facial perception (Pictures of Facial Affect PFA; Ekman 1993; with kind permission of Paul Ekman Group; www.paulekman.com)

tions are compared with each other. Features associated with different emotions are defined. For example, some participants often have difficulties distinguishing between fear and surprise or between anger and disgust.

Optionally, the participants can show the different basic emotions using their own facial expressions. Yet it is not recommended to request a participant directly to show a basic emotion. First, the connection should be made to participants' everyday lives.

Examples of Key Questions

- Is it easy for me to express my feelings in front of other people?
- Do I generally feel well understood?
- Do others react adequately to the feelings I express? For example, do they notice when I'm very happy about something?

Individual practice in emotional expression is supported (or provoked) by an external stimulus. A short, fictitious situation described by the primary therapist or a situation experienced by a participant can function as the stimulus. This didactic approach to promoting perception of one's own affective states and those of others is very activating in the group context. However, it requires a high level of structuring by the therapists. Participants with pronounced negative symptoms often exhibit considerable deficits in this (affect flattening). They should be positively reinforced and protected from excessively negative assessments and interpretations by other participants ("The intensity of the expression of emotion varies from person to person and depends on the situation"). Then again, other participants show considerable deficits in affect decoding, leading to misinterpretations. In this case, therapists introduce the same emotion recognition techniques based on facial features that were used when processing the standardized pictures (▶ CD Information Sheet 7: "How do I recognize the feelings of others?").

Affect Decoding Stage 2: Facial Expressions and Gestures

Building upon the recognition of emotions using facial features, the task is now to identify facial expressions and gestures on a higher performance level. This primary intention of this intervention unit is to raise awareness of observable nonverbal behavior for emotion recognition. In a group discussion, therapists introduce gestures as further ways to express emotion (▶ CD Information Sheet 8 "A gesture often says more than 1000 words"). The examples of gestures contained on ▶ CD Worksheet 8 and their meanings are discussed in the group and participant self-perception is promoted by asking about their own experiences. The information about gestures on ▶ CD Worksheet 8 is supplemented by participant comments. In addition, other emotional states are added to the basic emotions, shame and interest for example. This is followed by an exercise, the goal of which is recognizing and interpreting feelings using gestures and facial expressions.

For this, the nine photographs contained on the ▶ CD-ROM are used (▶ CD e-Materials 2a–i). These black-and-white photographs show the gestures and facial expres-

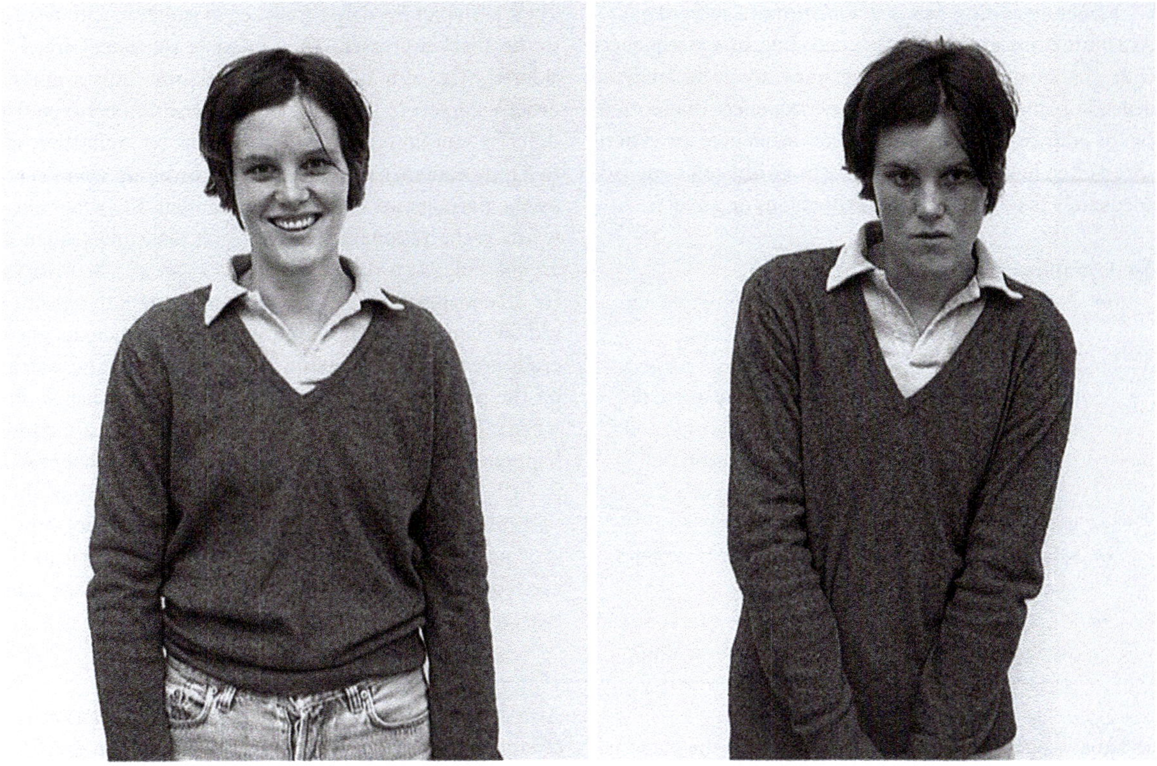

Fig. 2.9 Affect decoding stage 2: facial expressions and gestures (Hodel 1998; with kind permission of B. Hodel)

sions of a young woman for various emotional states (Fig. 2.9). In addition to the basic emotions, the emotional states of shame, interest, and physical pain are also depicted. An emotionally neutral image completes the series.

This series of pictures was evaluated using 100 healthy test persons (Hodel 1998): 28 men and 72 women between the ages of 15 and 51. The photographs were assessed using a multiple-choice method with the aforementioned categories as possible options with the exception of the category "neutral". Women tended to recognize the depicted target emotions somewhat better than men (exception: pleasure). Yet the difference was insignificant. Table 2.2 summarizes the results of correctly assessed emotions by the entire test population. The photograph with the emotionally neutral expression (▶ CD e-Materials 2i) was clinically tested but not taken into account for analysis.

The photos of emotions expressed by gestures are handled using the same procedure as the pictures of facial expressions. The participants are asked to identify the depicted emotions by means of facial expressions and gestures. Argumentation based on facts (features visible on the image) is encouraged; spontaneous assumptions and assertions are called into question. Therapists also point out the harmony of gestures and facial expressions when identifying the target emotion so as to create an overall view of nonverbal, emotional expression. Often, it is only after combining gestures and facial expressions into a unified image that some participants can recognize the target emotion.

Table 2.2 Evaluation of the picture series "Affect decoding stage 2": facial expressions and gestures ($n = 100$) (Hodel 1998)

Image number	Target emotion	Correct assessments (%)
e-2a	Pleasure	98
e-2b	Fear	76
e-2c	Anger/rage	77
e-2d	Disgust	75
e-2e	Grief	90
e-2f	Interest	96
e-2g	Shame	73
e-2h	Physical pain	68

Again, the gesture and facial expression accompanying an emotion can optionally be acted out in a role play and then discussed. This can help reconnect with the everyday life of the patients. This process, along with the risks involved, was described above (Affect Decoding Stage 1: Facial Perception).

Affect Decoding Stage 3: Emotional Sequences

As a more complex stage of affect decoding, image sequences with changing emotional expressions are now analyzed instead of single pictures. This way, sequences of emotions can be addressed in the therapy. Such sequences are experienced often in everyday life and are more difficult to decode adequately than isolated facial expressions or gestures.

Examples of Key Questions

- In everyday life, we are sometimes confronted with situations where the emotional states of our conversation partner changes in quick succession. For example, a person receives a gift. He or she first expresses surprise with their facial expression and gestures, followed by pleasure. After seeing the contents of the present, he or she might show annoyance. Have you observed such situations?
- Have you yourself ever been surprised at first, then glad, but ultimately annoyed?
- Recalling that situation, which of these emotions had the most impact on you and your conversation partner and has remained most in your memory?

The goal is again to establish a connection to the personal, everyday lives of the participants. ▶ CD Vignette 4 ("Rendezvous at a cafe"), which has already been discussed, can be used as an example of a possible sequence of emotions. It is important to point out to the group that this is not about stable states of emotion, such as long-lasting grief. The idea is rather that emotional states can change relatively quickly in connection with one's thoughts, behavior, and body perception, even within a single situation. Individual experiences contributed by the participants are again summarized on the flip chart.

For this intervention unit, further didactic material is also available on the accompanying ▶ CD-ROM (▶ CD e-Materials 3a–b: Emotion Perception Stage 3: Emotional Sequences). On each slide are 4 to 5 pictures of the same person with varying emotional expressions or no emotional expression. Each of these images is designated with a letter. The task is to put the pictures in the right order and to make an argument of why the suggested emotion sequence is the correct one.

Examples of Key Questions

- Imagine the pictures you are looking at are snapshots from a film. We don't know exactly what has taken place between the pictures in the film. Despite this, the pictures give us information with which we can get an idea how the film's plot might unfold. Specifically, each picture expresses a certain emotion. Which?
- Do you have a suggestion of which arrangement of pictures can explain the emotion sequence?
- Do alternative emotion sequences exist?

Thus, each picture is first analyzed in isolation with respect to the affect expressed. Then possible sequences are considered. The aim is to put the pictures into a correct order – correct in the sense of the transition between two different emotions (▶ CD e-Materials 3a: e.g., reflective, sad to happy, radiant). Every alternative ordering volunteered by the participants is first recorded neutrally. Only afterwards is the rationale given. Several plausible sequences are possible. As a rule, any sequence can also be reversed (▶ CD e-Materials 3a: e.g., from happy, radiant to reflective, sad). When giving their arguments, the participants generally are already employing ToM skills (e.g., "The woman on the pictures had a good day and was very happy. But when she thought about something or something happened, she became reflective. Happiness disappeared from her face. Her expression was neutral at first, then becoming increasingly reflective and finally melancholy."). This exercise thus also serves as an introduction to the concept of ToM and social perception, the social-cognitive target areas of Module B.

Emotional Concept Formation

As a final intervention in this target area, various ranges of emotion are introduced. Now the focus is on discriminating ranges of feeling with all their variations and nuances, which also manifest themselves in different concepts.

The card-sorting exercise "Terms of Emotion" is utilized for this purpose (▶ CD Materials 5a–h). Affective concepts are listed on a total of 97 small cards. Eight general terms, each designating a different range of feelings, are on the green cards. The ranges of feeling included here are the basic emotions defined above: fear, pleasure, disgust, grief, surprise, and anger. These are supplemented with love and self-confidence. The rest of the 89 cards are white and each contains a subordinate term for one of the green cards (◘ Fig. 2.10).

The 97 cards are distributed randomly. Each participant lays the cards they have received face-up on the table.

Examples of Key Questions

- Each of you has now received different cards. Do you notice anything? Do all the cards have the same color?
- We have now placed all 8 of the green cards in the middle. On the green cards are all the basic emotions we have defined as well as a couple of others. Can the white cards be assigned to these basic emotions? If yes, can you explain this assignment?

The participants now take turns assigning one of their white cards with subordinate terms to one of the green cards and justifies this (e.g., "When I'm happy, I also feel

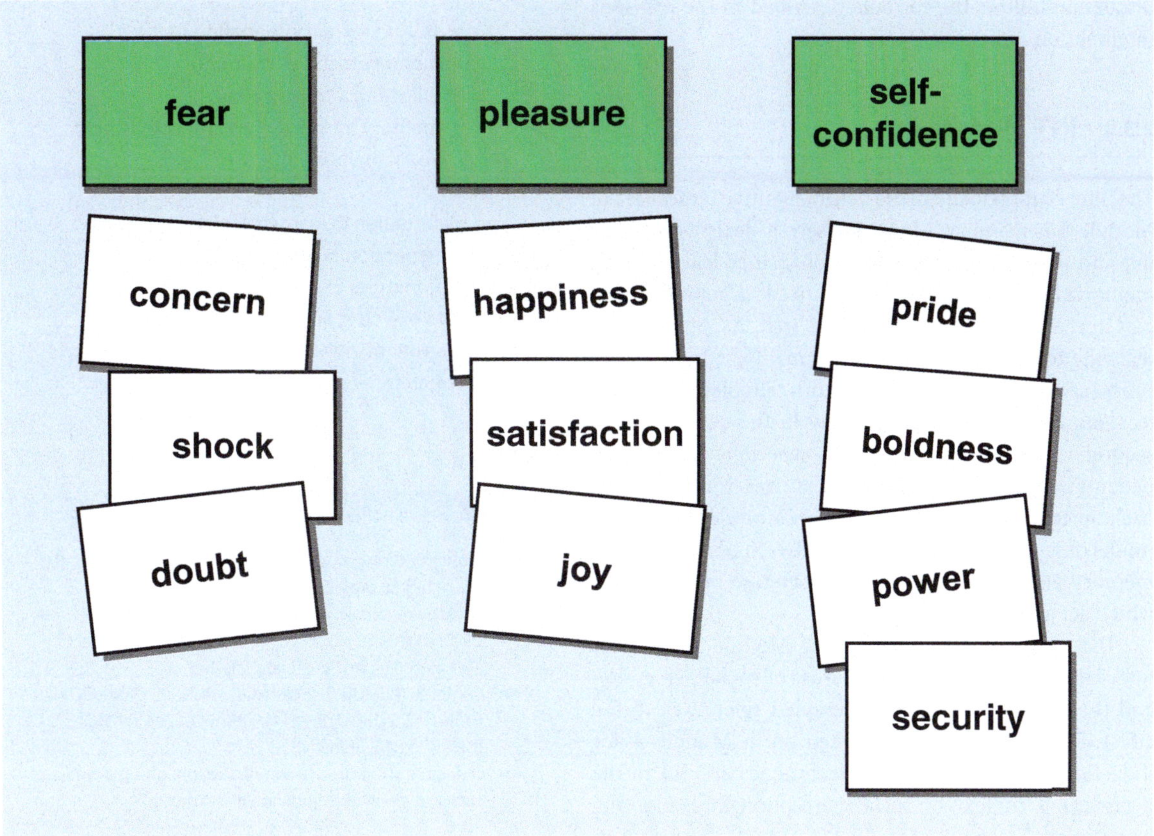

Fig. 2.10 Card-sorting exercise: "Terms of Emotion"

pleasure" or "When I'm brave, I also have self-confidence"). If one subordinate term is assigned to two different general terms and both lines of reasoning are plausible, the white card in question is put between the associated green cards. Once again, it is the participant's ability to make an argument which is at stake here, not a dichotomously right or wrong assessment. This card-sorting exercise is used again in Module C (Reasoning and Problem Solving).

2.3.1.2.3 Restitution

In the restitution section, newly learned strategies for affect decoding are now practiced repeatedly to the point of habituation. In terms of scope, stage 1 (affect decoding of facial expressions) takes up most of the restitution. However, for didactic reasons and to give variety to the sessions, therapists should continuously intersperse exercises from the 2nd stage (facial expressions and gestures) and 3rd stage (emotion sequences). Finally, each participant again assesses his or her current performance level with respect to emotion perception on ► CD Worksheet 6 ("How well can I recognize the feelings of others?"). Improvements in self-assessment compared to that made in the introductory section are discussed along with changes for the worse or stagnation. The latter are often an indication that the interventions are too demanding for those persons or that their motivation is not yet sufficient. Both situations should be addressed in one-on-one talks if required.

2.3.1.2.4 In Vivo Exercises and Independent Exercises

In social-cognitive target areas such as emotion perception, in vivo exercises often involve the risk of being too activating and too stressful for the participants. This is because they are based on social interaction. Thus, it is sometimes preferable to organize exercises on emotion perception so that participants experience them as passive observers. For example, the group can watch films together. The participants would then have the task of concentrating specifically on emotions expressed via facial expressions and gestures as well as identifying contradictions to the discussed text ("Nonverbal behavior never lies"). Such a joint activity requires thorough debriefing.

As an independent exercise, the participants can transfer such observer functions to their everyday lives. Prior to this, ► CD Worksheet 5 (independent exercise) should be filled out to prepare for the task. The subsequent discussion follows the formula described in the previous intervention unit.

2.3.2 INT Module B

The intervention focus in the neurocognitive target area of Module B is memory. More precisely, it deals with learning and memory as target functions, since learning and memorization techniques are practiced as coping strategies in the compensation section as well. As regards content, the topic is verbal and visual memory. In addition, prospective memory is introduced to supplement verbal learning and memory, particularly in the compensation section. Prospective memory is especially crucial for patients in order to lead independent lives. Module B falls back on content already addressed in Module A: the filter model describing the relationship between perception and memory and factors influencing cognitive performance, which act as filters.

The social-cognitive section of Module B contains interventions for the two target areas of social perception and theory of mind (ToM). Therapists refer back to the affect decoding techniques worked on in Module A for didactic purposes. Here, these techniques are put in the overarching context of social perception and adopting interpersonal perspectives (ToM). These interventions originated primarily from the subprogram "Social Perception" of Integrated Psychological Therapy (IPT) (Roder et al. 2008a, 2010).

2.3.2.1 Neurocognitive Intervention Area: Verbal and Visual Learning and Memory

Module B: Neurocognitive Intervention Area: Verbal and Visual Learning and Memory

1. Introduction
   - Definition of the target area: verbal and visual memory
   - Types and contents of memory: prospective memory
   - Self-perception in the target area (cognitive profile)
   - Reference to everyday life and self: case vignette
2. Compensation
   - Learning and individualizing coping strategies:
     - written memory aids
     - using the senses
     - memory tricks for enumerations
     - storing textual information
     - memory tricks for counting
     - following a conversation
     - memory tricks for keeping appointments
     - visual memory tricks
3. Restitution
   - Habituation of learned coping strategies:
     - Repetition of group exercises
     - Computer Exercises
4. In vivo exercises and independent exercises
   - Transfer of individualized coping strategies to concrete, everyday situations

Tips

- Infrastructure: group therapy and computer rooms, flip chart, digital projector
- Therapy materials: ► CD Information Sheets 6, 9–15, ► CD Worksheets 4–5, 7–10, ► CD Vignettes 5–8, ► CD Materials 6–8, ► CD e-Materials 4–5
- CogPack: MEMORY, NEWorNOT, ARCHIVE, ONtheROAD, EYEWITNESS, ROUTE, ALPHA-BRAVO, CAR-SYMBOLS, INHABITANTS, READING
- Didactics: structured group discussion, group exercises, computer exercises (individual and group)

2.3.2.1.1 Introductory Sessions

▪ **Definition of the Target Area: Verbal and Visual Memory**

As an introduction, the neurocognitive function "memory" is described. Therapists first point out the relevance of memory not only for everyday coping and planning but also for forming identity through stored experiences:

Introduction Example

In everyday life, we need memory in order to make a mental note of names, telephone numbers, birthdays, faces, or objects so that they can be recalled later. Yet memory encompasses much more than this. In a nutshell, our memory determines everything we know. All the experiences that have formed our character are stored in our memory. Memory represents the identity of a human being. Do you remember the filter model that you received as a handout? Whatever is stored in our memory also determines how we perceive things and how we react to them.

► CD Information Sheet 6 (Module A: filter model of perception) is briefly recapitulated in order to explain to the participants the connection between the function of memory and other cognitive functional areas. The factors influencing memory discussed in Module A (mood, emo-

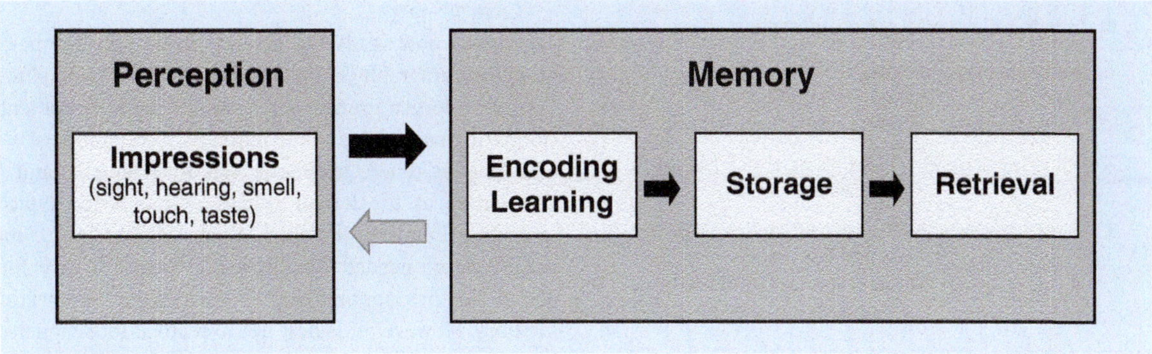

Fig. 2.11 Explanatory model: memory

tions, alertness, medications, etc.) can be illustrated using simple examples.

Example Exercise The participants are asked about an experience from the last 7 or 14 days that spontaneously comes to mind. As a rule, either particularly positive experiences (e.g., being invited to a good meal, the "right" team won in a football match) or particularly negative experiences (e.g., a fight, symptoms of illness) are mentioned. Based on these experiences, the group discusses the increase in memory performance in formative, emotion-triggering experiences.

Other influential factors such as alertness and daily rhythm or mood might also be briefly discussed. Yet depending on the group constellation, the negative effect of the consumption of substances like alcohol or cannabis on memory may be more relevant. The following questions might be used to expand on factors that affect memory:

Examples of Key Questions

- Is it equally easy for you to remember things in the morning, during the day, and in the evening?
- When you're in a bad mood, can you remember things just as well as when you're in a good mood?
- Do you think it's possible for someone who has consumed a lot of alcohol not to remember what happened anymore?

The objective is to increase awareness that these factors affect not only attention, but also the powers of perception and memory.

As a continuation of the filter model, the memory model (▶ CD e-Materials 4) is introduced to the group (Fig. 2.11). In addition to illustrating the interdependence between perception and memory, therapists should subdivide the memory process into encoding/learning, storage, and retrieval. This structuring serves as a basis for resource promotion and memory performance in the following compensation section. The focus of Module B is on learning and storing memory content. The ability to recall is first discussed in detail in Module D during the intervention on working memory.

Types of Memory

Because of the different types of memory and the varying use of the term "memory" in everyday language, it is difficult to find a basic, generally comprehensible usage for the following interventions. Usually, every participant claims to know what the power of memory entails. But are the differently applied types and features of memory all identical? The point is not to communicate specialized psychological knowledge about memory, but to define a common language. This standardizes participant knowledge and prepares it for later interventions. With the help of ▶ CD Information Sheet 9 (memory), the previously introduced model of memory is made available to participants as a source of information. The handout also indicates the distinction between short-term and long-term memory. The information sheet is introduced briefly by the primary therapist, read jointly section by section, and finally summarized by the group. The following is a possible introduction to the information sheet:

Introduction Example

When we remember what we have experienced, seen, heard, felt, or learned, it matters whether it took place 5 s (short-term memory) or 5 min (long-term memory) ago. (Module D distinguishes these types of memory from working memory as a control center and ultra short-term memory). Short-term memory has less capacity and the retention period is hardly longer than 20 s. If we retain something in our memory for a longer time, this is achieved by long-term memory. Yet in both short and long-term memory, the object is to encode or learn information, to store it, and then later to retrieve it for use in everyday life.

The co-therapist reads a simple word list of 20 words. This exercise aims to activate the participants and to illustrate the limited storage capacity of short-term memory. Examples can be found on the enclosed ▶ CD-ROM

Table 2.3 Categories of memory content

1.	Verbal learning and memory	Words Numbers (number series) Word lists
2.	Visual learning and memory	Faces, places, objects (visual and spatial-local memory)
3.	Prospective memory	Remembering future events that were agreed upon (appointments) or are fixed (e.g., birthdays)

(▶ CD Materials 6a–b). However, memorization techniques will first be discussed later in the next compensation section. In order to prevent social anxieties or fears of failure, this exercise is carried out in a group setting and together with at least two other participants. The goal is to recall memorized terms following a short distraction (e.g., solving a simple calculation).

Memory Content

To prepare for the memorization techniques (memory tricks) given in the compensation section and to complete the memory model, different types of memory content are summarized. For this, ▶ CD Information Sheet 10 ("Types of memory content") is available. For didactic purposes, a distinction is drawn between the following three categories of memory content (Table 2.3).

Therapists then point out that memory content is stored as a network. A word, number, face, or place is compared with previously stored content and thereby acquires meaning.

Example

For example, if you hear the familiar word "tiger", you immediately imagine something associated with it. You know that this is a really big and dangerous cat that lives in Asia. You can also make an internal image of this large cat since you have certainly already seen a tiger in a book, on TV, or in the zoo.

Promoting Self-Reference and Reference to Everyday Life in the Cognitive Target Area

Therapists relate the topic to patients' individual lives using the same didactic means as in Module A. The participants are first asked how they asses their own ability to remember the content listed on ▶ CD Information Sheet 10 ("Types of memory content"). If possible, they should describe related concrete experiences from their everyday lives. Participants generally underestimate their own powers of memory. Participant accounts regarding concrete situations are recorded on the flip chart. In addition, each participant fills out ▶ CD Worksheet 7 ("How good is my memory?").

Case Vignettes

The group now reads the case vignettes together paragraph by paragraph (▶ CD Vignettes 5–8). ▶ CD Vignette 5 ("A day to forget") summarizes various memory contents (forgetting names, telephone numbers, a shopping list). ▶ CD Vignettes 6 ("A telephone call for Daniel") and 7 ("Yesterday at the Italian restaurant") describe typical everyday situations in which short-term memory and retentivity are needed. Finally, ▶ CD Vignette 8 ("The forgotten doctor's appointment ") focuses on prospective memory. However, it is best not to read all four vignettes in one sitting. Most participants would not be able to absorb all the content at once. The first two vignettes can usually be read sequentially, however. ▶ CD Vignettes 7 and 8 can then be used to introduce the topic of coping strategies in the following compensation section.

After reading the ▶ CD Vignettes (7–8), a group discussion is held with the following goals:

- **Self-reference:** Participants make a connection to their own, personally experienced memory resources and deficits. There may be disagreement with plot of the vignette ("That's completely the opposite in my case").
- **Reference to everyday life:** Participants put the story in the context of their own experience and describe paradigmatic situations from their everyday lives.

The following questions are possible guidelines for therapists for structuring self-reflection on these two points:

Examples of Key Questions

- What can I remember well in everyday life? Names, conversations, and telephone numbers or persons, faces, and places?
- When and where do I have memory problems in everyday life?
- Where do I generally need such skills?
- Are there situations in everyday life in which my memory is especially good?
- Do the moods and emotions we discussed in past sessions play a role in my power of memory?
- What or whom do I remember especially well? What or whom especially poorly?

Other key questions on prospective memory:

- Where in my everyday life do I require the ability to remember appointed times like doctor appointments or birthdays?
- Is it easy for me to keep appointments?
- What aids do I use to remember appointments?

The group now explores individual, subjective experiences of strengths and weaknesses associated with memory in everyday life. In the process, therapists should establish a link to the social-cognitive sections of this module.

Perception and ensuing memory processes (encoding, storage, retrieval) should be put into concrete social contexts. As always in INT methodology, participant self-reflection is not reduced to disclosing personal deficits. Instead, resources are stressed. Therapists should also strive to make a participant's individual resources useful for the whole group:

Examples of Key Questions

- You have no difficulties with memory in this area. Can you tell us how you do that? Is there a memory trick you can reveal to us?
- You said that you are very pleased with your power to remember this type of content. Is that always the case? What does it depend on?

2.3.2.1.2 Compensation

The goal of the introductory section was to find a common language for concepts of memory and to support the participants in relating the types and content of memory to their everyday lives. This introduction simultaneously prepared the group for finding coping strategies, which is the aim of this section.

▪ Coping Strategies for Improving Memory

At the start of the session, the participants are asked which coping strategies, memorization techniques or memory tricks they know and already use in their everyday lives. Generally, participants repeat memory tricks already mentioned in the introductory sessions. As before, less promising examples are initially acknowledged without reservation. Each strategy mentioned is recorded on the flip chart together with the individually experienced situation in which the strategy was applied. This is followed by a group discussion focusing on the evidence of the strategies that were compiled. To prevent any participant from becoming insulted, statements such as "This strategy is useless" should be avoided. Instead, structured conversation elicits which of the strategies participants can imagine trying out, whether they think they are already capable of doing so, and what advantages they see in it. Several didactic supplements are available for this (▶ CD Information Sheets 11–15b).

▪ Written Memory Aids

As shown in the memory model (◘ Fig. 2.11), the storage process begins with the encoding or learning of perceived information. The group's first step towards optimizing memory performance is thus to discuss the function of understanding the information that is to be stored ("I must know and understand exactly what I should remember"). ▶ CD Information Sheet 11 ("Memory tricks: Inquire, repeat, and write down") is used as a didactic tool for this purpose. The techniques of requesting and repeating information are explored as ways to complete or check the correctness of that information. Writing down information as an external memory aid is also stressed. In addition, it can be highly beneficial in the everyday life to reduce the amount of information, and only taking note of information that is important for achieving the objective.

To illustrate the advantages of this memory trick, the following role play can be performed (◘ Fig. 2.12). It is not included on the ▶ CD-ROM since it should be adapted to regional conditions for the sake of the participants (excursion destination; train or bus connections).

▪▪ Exercise: Inquire, Repeat, and Write Down

Content The case vignette's protagonist Peter has decided to go on an excursion tomorrow by train. He has already chosen a destination (from Bern to the Jungfraujoch, home to the highest restaurant of the Alps, and thus also called the "Top of Europe"). He called the train information office to inquire about the exact route and departure times (the highly complicated and long itinerary is taken from the official Swiss timetable). However, the person providing the information is under stress and reads him the information rather quickly.

Objective In the role play, participants should try out asking for and writing down information.

Procedure

1. First, one participant is chosen for the role of Peter. The co-therapist assumes the role of the information person. Both receive a written copy of their text.
2. In the first run, Peter calls the information person without prior instruction or receiving a text. In the role of the information person, the co-therapist reads his or her text very quickly and then says goodbye, Peter will probably have stored little of the information.
3. The group discusses what information is important for Peter to reach his destination safely.
4. Starting with the 2nd run, participants practice how to interrupt the information person and how one can ask questions in order to write down the essential information regarding departure/changing times and platforms. Another participant can assume the role of the information person.
5. Each role play is discussed by the group extensively. Feedback is given in this order: the active actor (Peter), the passive actor (information person), the other group members (of whom some may have been assigned observer roles with concrete functions), and finally the therapists.

For further practice of limiting and storing pertinent information, the enclosed ▶ CD-ROM contains materials

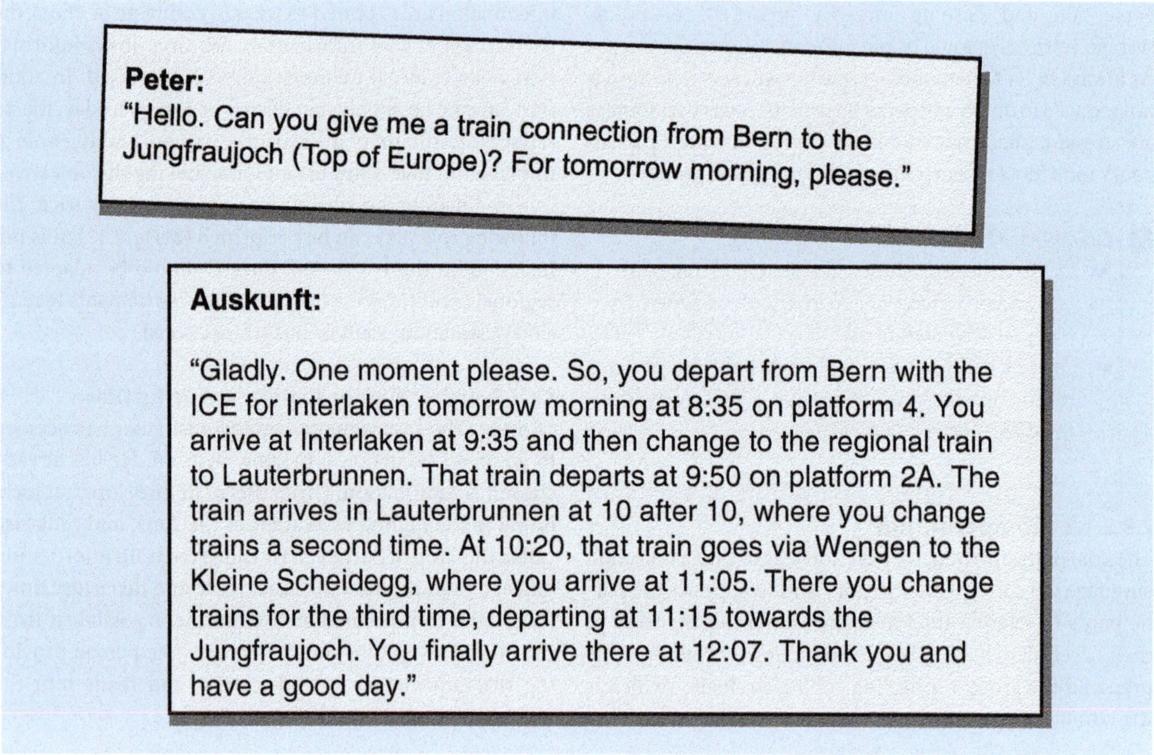

Fig. 2.12 Memory exercise: inquire, repeat, and write down

with short texts of typical everyday conversations (► CD Materials 7a–h):

Procedure In this exercise, one participant reads the others a text, e.g., a conversation at the family doctor's (Fig. 2.13). In the meantime, the others take notes. Then, with peer support, participants try to reproduce the most important information. At the end of each text, example questions are listed that aim at the essential content of the conversation.

Using the Senses as Memory Aids

Further memory aids can be summarized by the title "using the senses". This concept is a useful didactic tool for helping the participants learn different memory strategies using a single keyword. Primary focus is placed on sight, hearing, and to a lesser extent on the touch. Yet smell and taste should also be integrated as further sensory modalities. The following is an example exercise that can serve as an introductory illustration of sensory modalities. It should be explained by the primary therapist as follows:

Introductory Exercise

Imagine you are in the waiting room of your family doctor and meet a middle-aged man. He is elegantly dressed, uses an intense-smelling aftershave, and gives you a firm salutatory handshake. During conversation, he offers you a delicious chocolate from a precious confectionery box. He has introduced himself to you as Mr. Barthuber-Stiegelmayer. After meeting him, you'd like to remember him. Of course, you'd also like to remember his name. To imprint this rather difficult name in your mind, you can make use of all five senses:

1. **Hearing:** Repeat the name out loud or internally, or perhaps put it to a melody such as we often hear on the radio or in TV commercials.
2. **Sight:** Write the name down and read it several times. You can also associate the name in a mental image with the elegant clothing or with physical attributes of the person concerned. Or imagine the name written elegantly on a chalkboard.
3. **Physical sensation:** Associate the name with the firm handshake, which perhaps surprised you and hurt slightly.
4. **Smell:** Associate the name with the person's intense aftershave, which you didn't like because it was too overpowering.
5. **Taste:** Finally, the taste of the sweet chocolate can also serve as a memory aid; he offered you one, and you asked him why he was eating chocolates in the waiting room.

The topic of using the senses as a memory technique is summarized on ► CD Information Sheet 12 ("Memory tricks: using the senses"). This information sheet is read section by section in the group. Participants also carry out a short demonstration exercise for each of the techniques listed. Examples of this will be briefly described in the following:

A Visit to the Doctor

Julia is at the doctor's with a throat ache, coughing, and fever. He checked her heart and examined her throat.

Doctor: "Yes, you have caught quite a cold. But you're lucky. It's not tonsillitis yet. Keep in bed for the next few days. Then you'll be back on your
feet. I'm prescribing you a spray for your throat. Use it three times a day. And please don't eat or drink anything afterwards for half an hour."

Julia: "Fine. And what can I do against this horrible irritation in my throat?"

Doctor: "For that I'd better give you some cough medicine. Take it in the morning and in the afternoon. And for the evening I'm prescribing you these cough drops as well. Take them at night whenever you throat is
particularly irritated."

Julia: "Great. Thank you very much."

Doctor: "And if you don't feel better by Friday, please come back to my office. Get well soon!"

Questions:
1. What is Julia suffering from?
2. What medication is Julia receiving?
3. When should Julia take each medication?
4. What should she bear in mind when doing so?
5. When should Julia go back to the doctor's?

Fig. 2.13 Conversation examples

Repeating Information The behavioral experiment (on the phonological loop) derived from Baddeley (1986) is a good illustration of the limited capacity of short-term memory and the support potential of repetition as a memory aid. It is done in two steps:

1. First the group practices saying together the word "Coca-Cola" ("ze-bra" or another two or three-syllable word) quietly, repetitively, and rhythmically. Then the therapist reads out a word list (working material 6a–d). Rhythmic repetition of the word "Coca-Cola" prevents the participants from being able internally to repeat the words in the word list (preventing the phonological loop). Then therapists check how many words the participants could memorize.
2. In the second step, the therapist reads the participants another word list, but this time without rhythmic repetition of the word "Coca-Cola". This makes internal repetition (the phonological loop) possible. The group's memory performance should be higher here than in the first step of the experiment.

This experiment, originally conceived for the area of working memory, clearly exemplifies the supportive effect of repetition when learning concepts. It also makes plausible connections to participants' everyday experience.

Making a Mental Image For illustrative purposes, the group can perform the well-known exercise "packing a suitcase". One after the other, participants are asked to pack an object in a "mental suitcase". First they should try to recall previously packed items and imagine them arranged in their own room or apartment. After repeating previously named objects, the participant adds a new one. Therapists should make sure that less capable participants are not overwhelmed in the process. Whispering or hand signals should therefore not be discouraged. They are completely welcome and serve to promote group cohesion. Moreover, all participants have the right to sit their turn out. Depending on the size of the group, therapists can also participate in this exercise. If the participants are asked before the exercise how many objects they can commit to memory, they generally underestimate their power of memory considerably. Memorization performances of 20 to 25 items by some participants are not rare.

Associating Concepts with Body Parts or Objects Instead of moving house, this exercise concerns packing a suitcase in preparation for a trip. The key question is: "What do I need for a trip or a long weekend?" In asking this question, each person surveys his or her body, coat pockets, and handbag and considers what should be packed. One might proceed, for example, from top to bottom: a comb for the hair, soap for the face, a toothbrush and toothpaste for the mouth, sweater and coat for the body, a wallet and possibly passport in the coat pocket or handbag, and finally spare socks for the feet. Participants ask themselves how it feels to carry a thick wallet in their coat pocket (tight and uncomfortable), to wear a sweater (pleasantly warm or scratchy), or to comb their hair (painful when there's a knot). The more nonsensical or emotionally charged the association is the better the concept will be remembered.

▪ Memory Tricks for Enumerations and Shopping Lists

When coping with everyday life, the ability to store several concepts while learning, shopping, or in conversation is crucial. ▶ CD Information Sheet 13 ("Memory tricks for remembering several concepts") summarizes coping strategies for memorizing lists of concepts. These are again rehearsed in the group by means of simple exercises:

Summarizing Concepts in Categories to Reduce the Number of Items to Be Memorized ("Chunking") Usually, participants noticed when using the word lists on ▶ CD Materials 6a–c that the terms could be subsumed under one of two categories except for one term belonging to neither. When performing this exercise, participants usually recall the incompatible term easily. Again: the more striking a concept or association is, the higher the probability it will be remembered.

Associating Objects with Places The procedure is analogous to the "packing a suitcase" exercise described above.

Putting Concepts into a Coherent Story Participants often complain that creating a story from various concepts is both difficult and stressful. It is thus recommended that this is practiced repeatedly as a group, thereby benefitting from the resources of all the participants. A simple exercise lends itself for this: Each participant names a concept from one category (or several categories) (e.g., favorite pet, favorite food, favorite color). For example, the following pets could be involved: three dogs, two cats, aquarium fish, a budgie, and a hamster. The group now puts these together into a story (e.g., "Our neighbor's extremely brutal budgie is chasing our three big German shepherds. They run off, loudly barking, into the distance. In the process they stumble over two cats from next door, one of which has just gotten hold of Grandma's hamster while the other was trying to steal a fish from the aquarium. 'We were lucky,' the fish think to themselves, while the hamster waves and expresses his gratitude to the budgie.").

Form a Word from the Initial Letters of Concepts This exercise involves coping with the same difficulties as the previously described technique. For this reason, the same applies here: practice as a group. One example is described on ▶ CD Information Sheet 13.

▪ Storing Textual Information

Another aspect of memory that is relevant to everyday life is remembering texts, be it when reading a newspaper, a book, instructions, or written messages. This area is a continuation of the section "Concentration Problems when Reading" from Module A. Again, we are concerned with remembering both the crux of the text's content and important details that are relevant to the key message. If participants complain about difficulties remembering the content of a text, attentional deficits generally go hand in hand with deficits in verbal memory, since there functions are mutually dependent. As a consequence, the first tip here as in the aforementioned section of Module A is to highlight or underline important content ("We must first decide what is important before we can store it"). The actual key information is usually reduced to a few terms or, depending on the text, to numbers contained in it. The following group exercises are good for illustration:

Recognizing Important Text Content The therapists bring various newspapers or magazines along to the session. Each of these newspapers should contain news articles. One or two participants take a newspaper and look for an interesting story. They read the short article and summarize it for the rest of the group. If the exercise is done in teams of two, they must first agree on what the basic idea of the news article is. Markers or something similar are expressly permitted. The other group members then summarize the report they have heard in their own words. The two participants who gave the report now monitor whether their message was understood correctly and amend it if required. Finally, the story is read and the group checks to see if its content has been conveyed properly.

Remembering Important Details In this exercise, the participants are asked to think of a sentence containing two numbers (e.g., "Three cats are chasing after five mice." or "In the year 2020, I'll be 50 years old."). Then the participants quote their sentences one by one. If the group is large, the primary therapist can interrupt occasionally to ask a few participants which numbers a certain participant mentioned. In the case of smaller groups, the numbers can be elicited at the end instead.

Memory Tricks for Counting

Numbers and number series are also discussed as another type of memory content. For illustration, the following introductory exercises can be performed in the group.

Telephone Numbers The co-therapist first writes a telephone number on the flip chart. One number follows the other, without spaces or arrangements. For simplicity's sake, the number can start with the local area code or, to increase the level of difficulty, with the international code followed by the regional code. One participant reads out the number series. Then it is covered. The participants are asked to recall the number series after doing a simple calculation task as a distraction. As in most memory exercises, probably the first few and sometimes the last few figures are reproduced correctly. The strategy of combining figures ("chunking") into units of 2, 3, or 4 is also discussed and attempted in the second round. In order to establish a link to real life and increase participant motivation, telephone numbers of movie stars or well-known public personalities are used starting with the second round. Of course, participants should not be given private telephone numbers, but those of fan clubs or offices. In our experience, some participants could still remember the number 3 weeks later.

Number Lists As a supplementary exercise, the co-therapist can read aloud one of the number lists provided on the ▶ CD-ROM (▶ CD Materials 6e). Breaking down the number list into two categories and combining/relating similar numbers or number sequences are discussed as memorization aids.

To further introduce the subject, to promote self-reference, and to help find coping strategies, the following key questions can be addressed:

Examples of Key Questions

- Who finds it easier to remember words? Who finds numbers easier?
- When and in what situation was the last time you couldn't remember numbers or number series?
- What possible ways do you know of improving number memorization? Which ones have you already tried out?

As a rule, participants find remembering numbers more difficult than remembering words. Examples of situations and experiences with coping strategies are compiled on the flip chart. ▶ CD Information Sheet 14 ("Memory tricks for numbers") serves as a supplement to the coping strategies volunteered by the participants. Again, the techniques are tried out in the group to illustrate them more concretely.

Chunking/Reducing the Amount of Numbers The introductory exercises have already discussed subdividing single columns of numbers into units consisting of several figures.

Number-melody associations: This technique for aiding the memorization of telephone numbers, used in advertising, should first be demonstrated by the co-therapist. Because of the technique's high degree of activation, participants tend to be rather reticent when it comes to applying it.

Number-Word Associations The goal is to find everyday associations for a fictitious telephone number or a bank code (example: "Is anyone aware of a meaning of or a connection to the number 75 from their own environment?"). In addition, therapists point out that bank machines and (mobile) telephones assign three letters to each number. With a bit of imagination, a word can thus be formed from the number series. This technique is also practiced as a group using a telephone number or a bank code.

Number-Picture Associations The technique can also be illustrated as an activating group exercise. The participants assign each number from 0 to 9 to a concept. The example on ▶ CD Information Sheet 14 serves as the model for this. Birthdays or the street numbers of participants' residences are then substituted with the corresponding concepts and presented to the group. The other participants are then asked to translate these back into numbers.

Following a Conversation

Many participants complain that it is difficult to follow what the other person is saying in a conversation. This then leads to experiences of stress and a reduced sense of self-worth. The person ultimately avoids conversation, leading to social isolation. The role of memory in conversation differs from other situations because it places greater demands on the person: new information must be encoded within a short, limited time and then existing information must be retrieved that is appropriate to the social context. The cognitive flexibility needed for this will be extensively dealt with later in Module D of INT.

Coping strategies were already introduced at the conclusion of the topic of verbal memory in conversational situations. The new strategies on ▶ CD Information Sheets 11–14 are now practiced again in a highly structured group conversation. To this end, the conversation exercise "new identity" is carried out. This exercise contains aspects of real, everyday situations and thus differs from memory exercises under laboratory conditions (◻ Fig. 2.14).

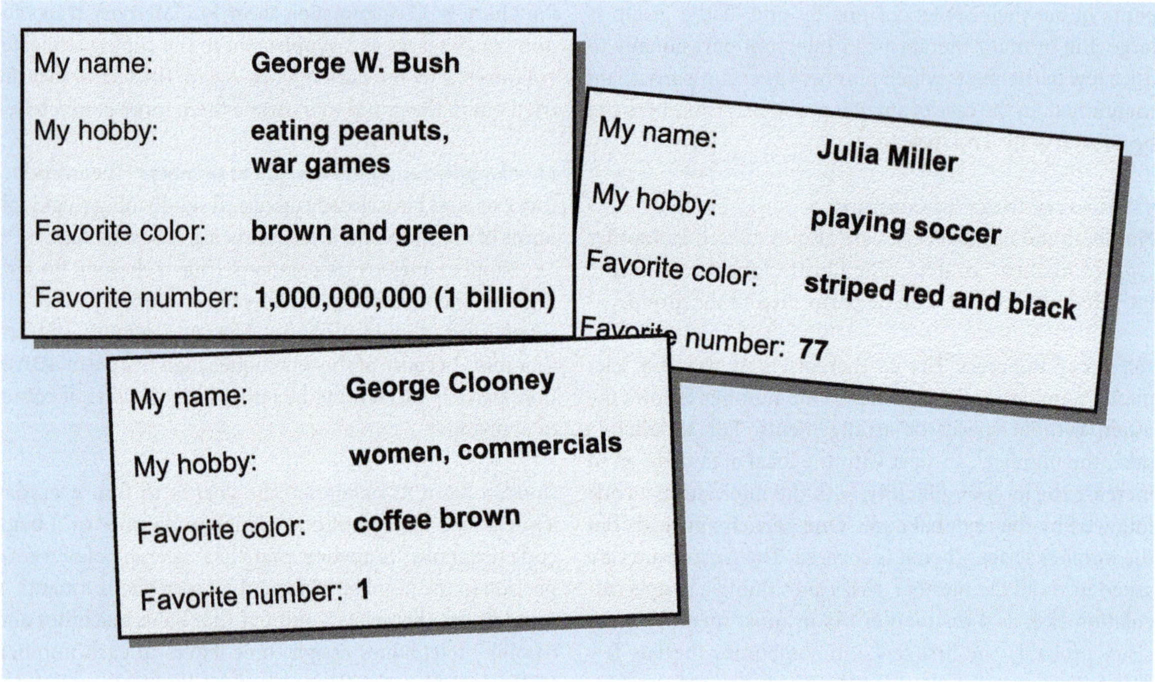

Fig. 2.14 Memory conversation exercise "New identity"

"New Identity" Each participant receives a card (► CD Materials 8a–b) on which are listed a person's name and a few features of that person (hobby, favorite color and number). The primary therapist briefly explains a social situation ("Imagine that complete strangers have gathered here and are now introducing each other…"). Following this, the primary therapist leads a highly structured group conversation, first asking each participant directly for his or her name (which is on the card). The primary therapist occasionally interrupts the round of introductions and asks one participant to remind him of the names of the members that have already been introduced (or the name of a particular group member). In the second round, each participant tells the group his or her hobby, in the third and fourth his or her favorite color and number. The primary therapist continues to interrupt and test the participants' memories. At the end of the exercise, the participants try to remember the entire personal description contained on each person's card. The object of this exercise is that the participants identify and each attempt to apply some of the coping strategies discussed. Of course, not every strategy is right for every participant, so each should develop his or her own individual repertoire of coping strategies. Finally, the group compares the varying levels of difficulty of the concepts that had to be memorized. For example, contradictory or illogical statements ("The favorite color of the football player Schweinsteiger of Bavaria is royal blue") and prominent names with expected hobbies ("George Clooney and women") are easier to recall than inconspicuous names ("Mr. Steingrau") or average hobbies ("family, cooking, gardening") unless one can relate these to oneself or someone close.

Memory Tricks for Keeping Appointments

If ► CD Vignette 8 ("The forgotten doctor's appointment") was not read already in the introductory section, this is a good opportunity to do so. Also, the following exercise is suitable for introducing prospective memory:

Introductory Exercise The primary therapist requests one of the group members who is wearing a watch to give a signal (e.g., in exactly 4 min) as then she will have something to say. While the primary therapist introduces the group to the topic, the corresponding participant gives a signal. As a rule, the signal is given exactly at the predetermined time. The participant is then asked how he or she was able to keep to the appointed time despite the group conversation. The most important reason will probably be that the participant in question continuously or repeatedly looked at the watch in order not to miss the time. Neighboring participants may have done so also. Thus, they used the watch like an agenda.

More precise coping strategies are summarized on ► CD Information Sheets 15a–b ("Memory tricks for appointments or future events"). The group discusses agendas, calendars, and bulletin boards as external memory aids.

However, there are always participants who do use external memory aids (e.g., an agenda or a mobile phone with an agenda function) and do take notes of appointments in them, but often still do not perceive them. The therapeutic goal in such cases is to adapt such implements to participants' individual daily structure. Also, therapists should provide incentive for improving their knowledge of and interaction with available tools. It should be clarified in advance what the reasons are for missing appointments and which coping strategies could be useful to counter them.

Memory Deficit Participants keep an agenda, but soon forget their appointments again. As a coping strategy, each participant stipulates at which fixed times every day the agenda will be consulted (e.g., after breakfast, after lunch, at 4 pm, and after dinner). As an additional coping strategy, the participants also learn to do the following the evening before or in the morning when they consult the agenda: They take a note on a piece of paper that they carry with them, on their hand as a cue, or on an easily visible paper hanging in their workplace or home.

Following an Agenda as Excessively Demanding Participants report that they do own an agenda but it is too demanding for them to enter and to retrieve all their appointments. They subjectively experience their appointments as being too copious. They constantly forget to enter appointments, misplace the agenda, or forget it at home. As a supplement to practicing keeping an agenda, it can be helpful for such participants to reduce the amount of appointments ("Which appointments are important?") or to limit the time frame to the following week. For this, ▶ CD Worksheet 8 ("My to-do list") and ▶ CD Worksheet 9 ("My weekly schedule") are available on the enclosed ▶ CD-ROM. On the to-do list, only appointments defined as important are included. The importance of various appointments can also be rated. The weekly plan reduces appointments to one calendar week and subdivides each day into morning, afternoon, and evening so that recreational appointments can also be included.

Avoidance Sometimes participants avoid (particular) appointments because they are associated with stress. In such cases, the causes of that stress have to be analyzed. What is at the root of such anxiety or unpleasant feeling? Are the (side) effects of a prescribed medication the cause of a "missed" doctor's appointment? Is being overtaxed at the workplace the real reason for an ignored appointment with the boss? Or is it (social) anxiety that lies behind a "forgotten" date? The stress caused by specific appointments often leads to a general avoidance of appointments and to social withdrawal. It is therefore important to clarify with the participant (in additional one-on-one conversations if required) whether thoughts and ideas associated with the stressful situation are realistic or whether they are the product of misinterpretations or delusional symptoms. As a rule, there are always other participants in the group who experience comparable stress and whose coping strategies can be utilized as resources. It may also be advisable in some cases to analyze the stress-inducing situation being avoided by means of the technique of cognitive restructuring and to develop alternative evaluations with the help of behavioral consequences. The aim is to guide such participants towards solution-oriented thought and action. Finally, therapists refer to the intervention areas of problem solving (Module C) and emotion regulation (Module D). In these, an (interpersonal) model for problem solving and techniques for coping with stress will be discussed.

It should be noted that some chronic outpatients exhibit few difficulties in prospective memory if the few, usually regular appointments that they have (e.g., medical visits or lunch with the family) provide them with a clear structure and stability in their everyday lives. These participants thus seldom forget such appointments. Therefore, if this area has little everyday relevance for the group, more space can be given to other INT treatment areas.

▪ Visual Memory Tricks

In conclusion, the topic of visual memory is addressed, which will be given greater weight in the following restitution section. The primary therapist introduces the topic of visual memory using everyday examples.

Example

In our everyday lives, sometimes we are forced to remember things visually, not with words. Here's an example of this: we are driving in an acquaintance's car to a shopping center and park the car. We each take care of various things in the shopping center. A certain time had been set to meet at the car on the huge and completely full parking lot. Now we're forced to remember our acquaintance's vehicle exactly so that we wait at the right place among all the parked cars. That means we will have had to memorize the features of the acquaintance's vehicle (size, color, etc.) as well as approximately where it was parked. This is referred to as visual and local memory.

This topic is directly affiliated with the techniques of verbal memory as well as the techniques of perceiving emotions and attention activation from Module A.

- **Focusing attention:** We must force ourselves to focus on the object to be remembered or its characteristic features ("I now want to remember this object and its features").
- **Making a mental image:** The participants imagine the object with closed eyes, associate it in their "inner" eye with other objects or with objects or places already known from their own experience.

- **Describing the object:** Like the facial features of an emotional expression in emotion recognition, here we focus on detailed description of the object's properties. In other words, the object's properties are translated into words: for example, shape, color, design, associations to well-known objects that we are already aware of, etc.
- **Categorizing objects:** If one has to commit several objects to memory, it is advantageous to combine these objects by means of their features: for example, round, angular objects, objects with the same color and size, etc.
- **Local description:** Not only the features of the object serve as memory aids, but also the position and surroundings of the object, i.e., its local features. Among other occasions, this technique is applied when a city map or a traveled route has to be learned in order to find the way back. Here, we are dealing with a sequence of different local descriptions.

Various exercises are possible to illustrate these techniques. Two exercises using therapy materials already mentioned will be described in the following:

Remembering Cards Either the cards from the IPT card-sorting exercise described in Module A (▶ CD Materials 1) or those of the card-sorting exercise "speed" (▶ CD Materials 2a–l) are used as stimuli. The primary therapist lays down several cards from one of the two card series for all the participants in an easily visible way. After a few seconds, the therapist covers the cards (with a large sheet of paper). The participants are now asked which cards they can remember. Before the second run, relevant memory strategies should be explained again so the participants can apply them. For example, all the yellow cards, all cards with round features, all cards on the lower edge of the table, all cards that together look like…, etc. can be combined. The exercise's level of difficulty can be varied by changing the number of cards presented and the interval allowed for memorization.

Memorizing and Marking Routes City maps and maps of subway networks and hiking paths are available for a further demonstration exercise (▶ CD e-Materials 5a–x): the participants must first memorize the given route (1st figure) and then mark it (2nd figure). In order to give each participant the chance to mark the memorized route individually before solving the task together as a group, a worksheet is also available for each city map (without route) (▶ CD Worksheets 10a–l).

2.3.2.1.3 Restitution

In this target area, restitution encompasses both the re-use of group exercises described already in the compensation section as well as the repeated practice of various computer-based exercises. The following will first describe the group exercises and then the computer-based exercises. In order to promote a conscious and goal-oriented application of individually selected coping strategies, each participant fills out ▶ CD Worksheet 4 ("My helpful strategies for …") before attempting an exercise pertaining to a memory area. On it, individually selected coping strategies are noted down and then evaluated upon completion of the exercises. The didactic use of ▶ CD Worksheet 4 has already been described in detail in Module A.

Group Exercises

The following group exercises, which have already been discussed, are recommended for repeated use:

Group Exercises

- Verbal memory: conversation
  - Texts with examples of everyday conversations (▶ CD Materials 7a–h)
  - Exercise "packing a suitcase"
- Verbal memory: enumerations and shipping lists
  - Remembering lists of concepts and names (▶ CD Materials 6a–d)
  - Putting concepts into a coherent story
  - Form a word from the initial letters of concepts
- Verbal memory: storing textual information
  - Storing short newspaper texts
  - Remembering important details of a text
- Verbal memory: memorizing numbers
  - Memorizing lists of numbers (▶ CD Material 6e)
- Verbal memory: following a conversation
  - Exercise: "new identity" (▶ CD Material 8a–b): the individual cards should be remade for this purpose. E.g. the participants are asked to write their favorite movie star, that star's best movie, estimated age and presumed place of residence on an empty card. Other examples are top athletes, politicians, or participants' neighbors. The procedure follows that described in the compensation section.
- Visual memory
  - IPT card-sorting exercise (▶ CD Materials 1)
  - Card-sorting exercise "speed" (▶ CD Materials 2a–l)
  - City maps, subway networks, hiking paths (▶ CD e-Materials 5a–x; ▶ CD Worksheets 10a–l)

▪ Computer-Based Exercises

The procedure follows the principles of "errorless learning" described in Module A. In the following, CogPack exercises associated with the topic will be described. Again, a separate computer is available to each participant ideally. The exercises are repeated individually. However, some of the computer exercises are done as a group. In these cases, the exercise is projected, and the group solves it together. Competitive exercises are also provided to activate and motivate the participants. In these, half of the group competes with the other half. The evaluation criteria are: which team answered the fastest, made fewer mistakes, could remember more, or worked faster. The following well-tried CogPack exercises are available:

MEMORY This typical memory exercise consists of 17 sub-exercises of different types of memory. The following exercises are recommended:

- **Verbal memory**
  - **"Words item by item" (exercise g) and "Shopping list items" (exercise h):** The objective here is to remember ten successive words, which then have to be typed in. This exercise requires that the participants use the computer keyboard for typing. If any of the participants are susceptible to typing errors, therapists assess the terms that have been remembered correctly but typed incorrectly as "correct". To activate the participants, these exercises can also be performed in the group or as a competition between two subgroups. The group is then split in half, and a digital projector is used. In the first round, the first team tries together to recall the concepts presented; in the next round, the second team does the same. The therapist types the words. The group that correctly remembered more words wins.
  - **"Shopping list 1 page" (exercise i) and "Names 1 page" (exercise j):** In 2 min, a shopping list of 20 items or list of ten names is presented. Then the participants have to type in the items/names they remember. The therapeutic method is analogous to that described above.
  - **"Names 4 pack":** Four names must be remembered. After a pause of 10 s, 12 names are shown. The original four must be identified by mouse click.
  - **"Words spoken" (exercise p) and "Shopping spoken" (exercise q):** Ten words are spoken by a computer-generated voice and must then be reproduced. Because of its acoustic presentation, these two exercises are more suitable as group exercises or team competitions. The method follows that described above.
- **Visual memory**
  - **"Traffic 6 pack" (exercise l) and "Flags 6 pack" (exercise m):** Four traffic signs must be remembered. After a pause of 10 s, 12 items are shown. The original six must be identified by mouse click.
  - **"Forms 3 pack" (exercise n) and "Patterns 4 pack" (exercise o):** Three forms or four patterns must be recognized among 12 similar items after 10 s.

The first six sub-exercises (exercises a-f) are suitable only to a limited extent since they expect memory recall after a pause or distraction (e.g., a calculation task of 1–3 min); after the entire sequence is completed, some also ask for an address given at the start of the exercise. These exercises are hardly consistent with the "errorless learning" approach and usually overstrain some of the participants. For this reason, these exercises are only recommended for participants with excellent memories.

NEWorNOT This exercise includes 20 sub-exercises (exercises a-t), in which 20–40 stimuli are presented in succession. The object is to press a key when a stimulus has already been shown once before. With the exception of "Names" (exercise q), all sub-exercises are focused on visual memory. Because they involve very similar stimuli or moving, flickering lines, the two sub-exercises "Patterns" (exercise p) and "Chaos graphics" (exercise o) are more difficult and can lead to visual strain or sensory overload for some participants.

ARCHIVE These exercises link visual and verbal memory. Participants must assign an individually chosen name or number to each picture in a series of successively displayed photos. The pictures are then shown again in a different order. The participants are asked which name or number they have assigned to the corresponding picture.

ONtheROAD The content of this usually very popular exercise overlaps with the intervention area of working memory (Module C). However, it makes a welcome change in the restitution section on verbal and visual memory (as does the exercise EYEWITNESS below). Like a computer game, the user takes the perspective of a driver, who encounters various traffic signs and vehicles on the way. Questions are then asked such as "What speed is allowed?" or "How many vehicles did you see?". A few possible answers are given (multiple-choice).

EYEWITNESS Like the exercise described above, the exercise EYEWITNESS is based on pictures in motion. An urban street scene is shown with honking cars, advertisements flashing on buildings, etc. The stimuli that should be remembered are presented visually, in writing, and acoustically. Afterwards, the program quizzes the user about details from the scene in multiple-choice format.

ROUTE The first 5 sub-exercises (exercises a-e) are comparable to the exercise "city map" (▶ CD e-Materials 5a–x; ▶ CD Worksheets 10a–n). But now the level of abstraction is higher. All the streets are ordered symmetrically. The participant must travel a previously shown route from memory. The last two exercises (exercises f-g: "shortest way") can be considered visual memory exercises only to a limited extent. They are more suitable for practicing problem solving, as is done in Module C.

ALPHA-BRAVO In the three sub-exercises on verbal learning and memory, each letter of the alphabet is assigned a word with the same initial letter. These letter/word combinations are learned via a spelling chart and then tested.

CAR-SYMBOLS Like the exercise ALPHA-BRAVO, car symbols from different countries are learned from a list and then queried individually.

INHABITANTS The sub-exercises (exercises a-h), eight in total, focus on remembering numbers.

READING The 9 sub-exercises (exercises a-j) deal with remembering texts. First a text is read. Then questions regarding details of the text are posed (multiple-choice). Because some technical and mathematical terms are used, the three sub-exercises on cooking recipes (exercise b-d) are more suitable for use with schizophrenia patients.

The other CogPack memory exercises (WISDOM, CALORIES, VOCABULARY) are either too challenging for schizophrenia patients or contain words from foreign languages. Therefore, use of these exercises can only be recommended for participants with relevant knowledge.

The optimal duration of exercises in the area of verbal and visual memory is generally shorter than those in other functional areas. In order to avoid overtaxing the participants, it is recommended that memory exercises be carried out less than 30 min at a time. As described in Module A, a round of targeted feedback follows each exercise sequence in the group room. The group discusses and summarizes their self-assessment of memory performance as well as the more or less successful application of individual coping strategies previously recorded on ▶ CD Worksheet 4. The therapists reinforce experiences of success and patient resources. If participants were not very successful, new coping strategies are sought that can be applied in the next computer session. At the conclusion of the restitution section, participants check and correct the performance assessments they made of their own powers of memory at the beginning of Module D on ▶ CD Worksheet 7 ("How good is my memory?"). If required, they also take notes of changes in this functional area.

2.3.2.1.4 In Vivo Exercises and Independent Exercises

The overarching objective of this INT intervention is that the participants apply newly learned compensation strategies for optimizing memory in their everyday lives. To supplement the practice of individually selected strategies in the restitution section, participants now do in vivo and independent exercises.

The independent exercises take into account the examples volunteered by the participants of difficulties and resources they have experienced in their everyday lives. To prepare for the independent exercises, each member of the group first fills out ▶ CD Worksheet 5 (independent exercise). The independent exercise should be planned individually in concrete steps. The topic of the independent exercise is described with a title. The concrete situation to be expected and the strategy to be employed are defined, and expected or feared difficulties are anticipated. In the following session, the results of the independent exercises are discussed extensively following these points. Possible independent exercises for the area of memory include:

- Asking specific questions at the next doctor's appointment, repeating important information internally, making a mental image, taking notes like the doctor
- Breaking a shopping list down into categories; in case of small purchases, trying to do without a shopping list and to remember the items in the context of a story
- Trying to read an interesting book or a long magazine article while taking notes or highlighting selections of the text
- Remembering names using the mnemonics mentioned above, e.g., memorize the first and last names of neighbors, coworkers, or the last names of other group member for the next session
- Using words to describe and categorize objects or persons that should be recognized in social contexts or at work
- Translating new or known telephone numbers into words
- Keeping an agenda and consulting it three times a day; additionally, using a bulletin board or hanging up a paper with important appointments and information

In addition to independent exercises, in vivo exercises with the group can be performed using the above examples.

The amount of stress caused by the target situation should be kept as low as possible; later it can be gradually increased. The stress level is usually highest in social interactions with emotional involvement or in cases of sensory overload. The following is an example of an in vivo exercise aimed at memory:

Bus Excursion The INT group resolves to take a short excursion by bus to a nearby park and to drink a coffee there in the park restaurant. First the bus schedule is studied: "When are the departure and return times?" (memorizing numbers). During the bus ride, those sitting next to each other have a conversation (being able to follow a conversation). On the street that passes the park, participants note whether a car of a previously determined brand drives by and how many other cars drive by (visual memory, number memory). In the self-service park restaurant, two participants are chosen to take the order of all the participants and therapists and to pick up the food and drinks at the counter (categorizing lists of terms). Finally, the group is asked whether someone can remember when the bus will drive back to the clinic. Every in vivo exercise concludes with a discussion. This is done immediately afterwards or in the next session.

2.3.2.2 Social-Cognitive Intervention Area: Social Perception

Module B: Social-Cognitive Intervention Area: Social Perception (Theory of Mind)

1. Introduction
   - Definition: social perception and perspective adoption
   - Self-perception in the target area
   - Resource-oriented individual profile in the target area
   - Connection to self and everyday life: case vignette
2. Compensation
   - Learning coping strategies for social perception-in 3 steps: collecting information, interpreting, finding a title
   - Adopting another person's perspective
3. Restitution
   - Habituation of learned coping strategies in repeated group exercises
4. In vivo exercises and independent exercises
   - Transfer of individualized coping strategies to concrete, everyday situations

Tips

- Infrastructure: group therapy room, flip chart, projector
- Therapy materials: ► CD Information Sheets 6–8, 16–19, ► CD Worksheets 4–5, 11, ► CD Vignettes 9–10, IPT picture series (► CD Materials 9a–g), cards: sets on perspective adoption (► CD Materials 10a–c), ► CD e-Materials 6; commercially available videos
- Didactics: structured group discussion

2.3.2.2.1 Introductory Sessions

▪ Definition of the Target Area

The interventions concerning the social-cognitive functions of social perspective and theory of mind (ToM) will be referred to as "adopting perspectives" in the following for the sake of better participant comprehensibility. These interventions build directly upon the emotion perception skills acquired in Module A. Emotional expression is now put in the overarching context of conversation or social action. Conceptually, social perception differs from emotion perception in this way: Here, the core meaning (relevant to the observer) of a social situation taken as a whole must be immediately recognized and correctly assessed. Interpretation of the emotional expressions of involved persons contributes to the interpretation of the situation. In the group topic of perception and interpretation of social stimuli, the INT method also introduces the concept of perspective adoption. "Putting ourselves in another's shoes", "knowing or assuming what others are thinking", and "what does this trigger in ourselves" – these all directly reflect the cognitive distortions underlying psychotic symptoms that often also exist in the case of stable schizophrenia patients. Summing up, the interventions on social interventions, now somewhat less structured, also include interventions on emotional perception and perspective adoption.

As presented in the filter model of perception (► CD Information Sheet 6) in Module A, perception is affected by individual memory experiences. The social-cognitive intervention area of Module B on social perception is based directly on previously acquired skills in the neurocognitive area of verbal and visual memory. In this way, the intervention is both didactic and easily understandable for the participants.

First, the group revisits previous therapy concepts. These are illustrated using a concrete example:

2

Introduction Example

During the last few sessions, we've been dealing with memory and with strategies for making better use of our memory. Before that, we discussed the perception of feelings. We learned from the filter model (▶ CD Information Sheet 6) that our perception and memory influence each other. Now we will turn to the role of perception and memory in social situations. How and what we perceive in the social situation of a conversation can include the feelings and thoughts expressed by others and ourselves, objects, and the place where the conversation is happening. These in turn determine what we remember later. Let's take our group as an example, just as we are experiencing it here and now: Look around and observe the furniture in the group room, the other participants, and the group leader. Consider what is central and most important for you and for others. How did you orient yourself? Is it the computer or the table that you like the most? Is it the emotional expression of other participants? Or the personal experiences you made during recent group sessions? It is possible for you to assess what other people in the group room are thinking right now or were thinking? So the key question is: What does each of us perceive in this social situation?

Participant contributions are summarized and recorded on the flip chart. Then the concept of social perception is defined. For this purpose, ▶ CD Information Sheet 16 ("Perceiving a situation") is available on the accompanying ▶ CD-ROM. On it, basic social perception processes are summarized, e.g., joining diverse bits of information contained in a social situation into an overall picture (◘ Fig. 2.15).

Definition Example

When we see a situation or a photograph of a situation with several persons and want to know exactly what is happening, we need the skill of social perception. That is, we have to put ourselves in the situation in order to recognize what happened between the persons concerned. This is very important in everyday life when we intend to take part in a conversation or in an action. This requires the same skills as when we turn on the TV too late or walk into a cinema and miss the beginning of the film. We first need to orient ourselves . We need to get an idea as soon as possible of what is happening in the film and what has already been shown so we can follow the plot. For orientation, we use dialog ("Who is saying what?"), places and props visible in the background ("Where is this taking place?"), and feelings that are being expressed ("What relationship do the characters have? What have they just experienced?"). In the process, we try to put ourselves in the characters' shoes so we can find out why a character is saying or doing something in particular in the current situation ("What do I think the others (characters) are thinking and feeling right now?"). In a good film with good actors, the director's conscious intention is to assist us in this (◘ Fig. 2.15).

▪ Promoting Self-Perception in the Cognitive Target Area

Participants are each asked how they assess their own ability to orient themselves in a social situation and to recognize the essential aspects of it.

Examples of Key Questions

Have you experienced following examples in your everyday life?

- When I see a photo in a newspaper or a painting in a museum of a social situation, do I immediately recognize what the picture is saying? Does it make a difference whether only one or two persons are depicted or a large group of people?
- Say I have arranged to meet friends, arrive a bit late, and my friends are already deep in conversation. Do I find it difficult to find out what they are talking about? What feelings does such a situation trigger in me? Does it make a difference whether only two or a group of friends are talking together?
- When I come home, turn on the TV, and start watching a film that has already started, can I follow the plot well? Do I quickly pick up on what happened before in the film when I wasn't watching? Do I give myself time until I have learned more about the plot, or do I usually change channels right away?
- When someone is telling me something and shows emotion while doing so – starts crying, for example – is it easy for me to empathize with this person so I can understand why that person is crying at the moment?

When referring to everyday experiences, participants may object that social perception is especially difficult in situations involving complex stimuli or a large number or persons; such situations are therefore avoided. If this happens, the therapists should first refer to Module D. In it, the INT program concludes with a discussion of selective attention. Also, in the social-cognitive section of Module D, participants learn techniques of emotion regulation and coping with stress resulting from sensory overload.

In addition, each participant now fills out ▶ CD Worksheet 11 ("How well can I recognize what is happening in a situation or a conversation?"). This worksheet is discussed in the same way as described above.

▪ Case Vignette

There are two case vignettes concerning social perception and perspective adoption on the enclosed ▶ CD-ROM: ▶ CD Vignette 9 ("Art opening") and ▶ CD Vignette 10 ("Back at Café Adonis"). The vignettes are read section by section as described above. The participants are then asked whether they have had similar experiences in their

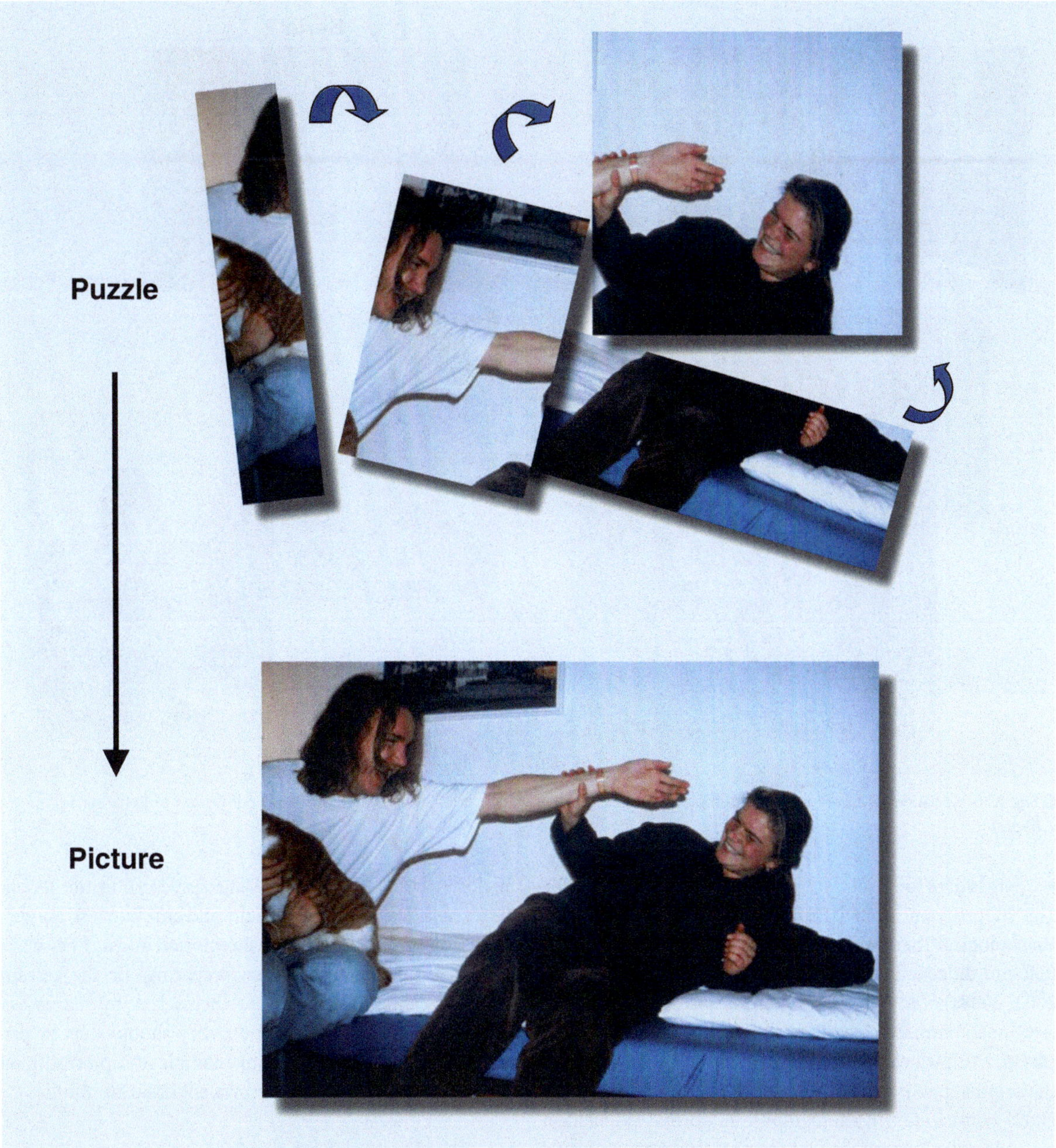

Fig. 2.15 Social perception: making an overall picture from various parts (Photos: V. Roder)

everyday lives. Again, the contributions of the participants are recorded on the flip chart.

▶ CD Vignette 9 is aimed primarily at self-reference in the area of social perception. It deals with the distinction between objectively existing facts (stimuli) and subjective assumptions. It thus also serves as an introduction to later exercises on perceiving and interpreting stimuli. ▶ CD Vignette 10 also focuses on the function of perspective adoption. It shows various criteria by which the protagonist Peter can orient himself in deciding whether and how to speak to Maria. Didactically speaking, ▶ CD Vignette 10 can thus be used both to relate the content to the participants' everyday lives and to introduce the following compensation section.

2.3.2.2.2 Compensation

Building on the introductory section, the group now develops coping strategies for improving the social-cognitive skills of social perception and perspective adoption. Participants will be given the opportunity to try out strategies in group exercises. The objective is that the participants build up individual repertories of coping strategies.

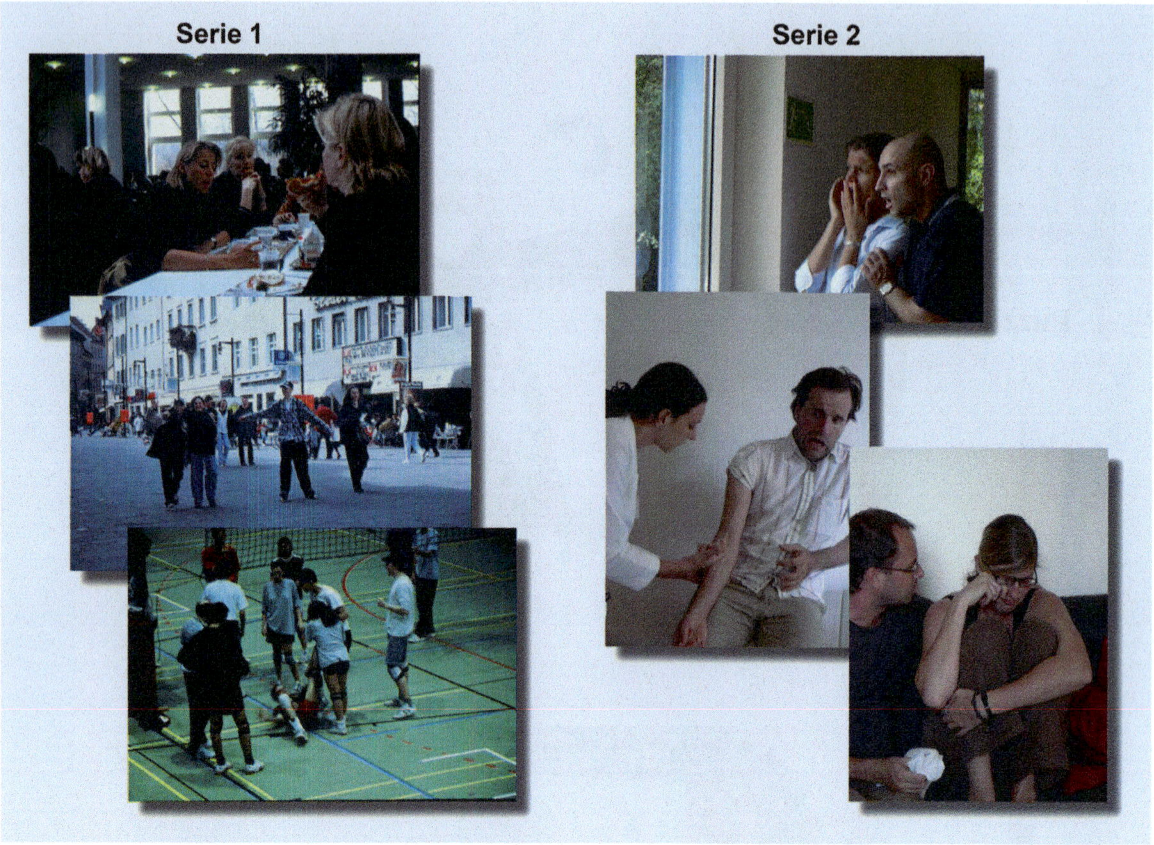

Fig. 2.16 Social perception: examples from picture series 1 and 2 (Roder et al. 2002, 2008a; with kind permission of Beltz Verlag, photos: V. Roder)

▪ Strategies for Social Perception

The subprogram "Social Perception" from the Integrated Psychological Therapy program (IPT) serves as the conceptual and didactic foundation for this section (Roder et al. 2002, 2008a). The IPT subprogram is based essentially on two standardized, well-established picture series (Fig. 2.16), which can also be used here and obtained by the original publisher. The first series of slides (Roder et al. 2002) consists of 40 photographs. A normal population assessed the photographs with respect to degree of visual complexity, emotional stress, and their titles. The title summarizes the content concisely. These assessments are listed on the ▸ CD-ROM (▸ CD Materials 9a–c) and provide the therapist with a basis for picture selection. It is best to start with less complex and less emotionally stressful images. The first slide series (method described below) is followed by the second slide series (Roder et al. 2008a), also consisting of 40 pictures. The latter series differs from the first insofar as it focuses more on representing social interactions. This gives more weight to the emotional expression of the persons depicted and also represents a continuation of the images used in Module A for affect decoding. Again, the assessments of the normal population are listed on the enclosed ▸ CD-ROM (▸ CD Materials 9d–g). In the second series of slides, cognitive capacity and emotional stress were assessed in addition to the basic emotion and a concise title for the image content. When preparing for the session, therapists should again orient themselves by the assessments of the normal population; they should start by presenting photos of lower cognitive complexity and emotional stress depicting clear, non-ambivalent basic emotions.

▪ Distinguishing Between Facts and Assumptions

First the participants are sensitized to the difference between facts and assumptions. Both are of central importance when interpreting a social situation. Referring back to the filter and memory model (▸ CD Information Sheets 6 and 9), the group discusses the influence of personal experiences on the perception process. The following simple, well-known, and usually activating introductory exercise is ideal for illustrating how we are directly influenced by our own experiences within a very short time period.

Introductory Exercise

The primary therapist speaks directly to a participant: "I will now mention a few concepts to you. You will then make a mental

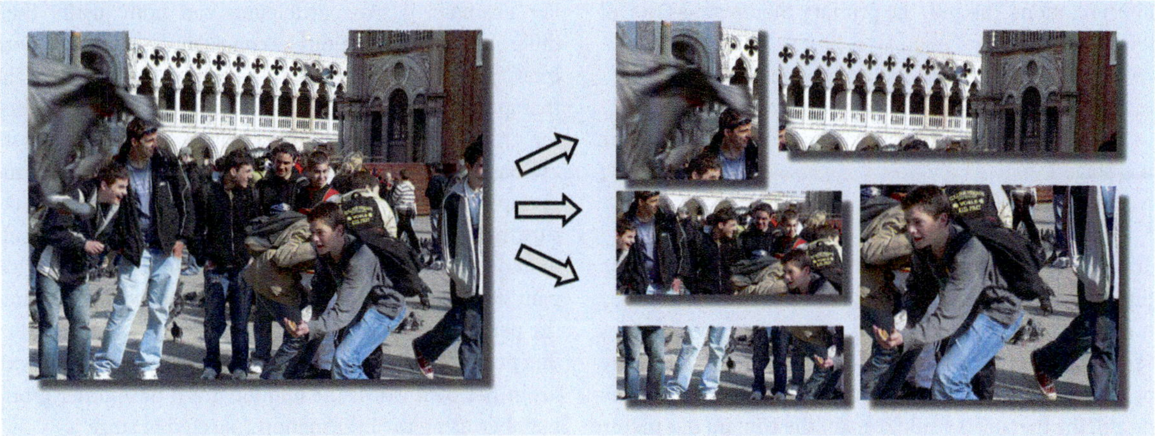

Fig. 2.17 Social perception: focusing on picture segments during information collection (Photos: V. Roder)

image of these concepts and tell me what color you see. What color is my (white) shirt?" "White!" "What color is the printed information sheet in front of you?" "White!" "What color is snow?" "White!" "What color is milk?" "White!" "What color is the cow the milk comes from?" "White…" Most test persons answer the last question the same way. If the person unexpectedly does not do this, the group is asked who would have given the answer "white".

The distinction between facts and assumptions is then explored further using ▶ CD Information Sheet 17 ("Assumptions are not the same as facts"). A picture from picture series 1 (Roder et al. 2002) is shown on it. When interpreting it, these two hypotheses emerge in many groups: that the man is pointing (a) out the window (to a car or a bird flying by) or (b) to the television (which is playing a football game, in which a goal or foul is taking place). The associated parties are then asked to support their arguments with facts (i.e., the light source, the facial expression of the woman, etc.).

Social Perception in Three Steps

The group works through the pictures of both series in three stages:

1. Collecting information
2. Interpretation and discussion
3. Finding a title

It is expressly recommended that therapists adhere to this three-stage sequence precisely. If the group starts interpreting too early (i.e., already in the information phase), the participants might overlook important information in their interpretations. This information will be missing from the discussion as a basis for argumentation. In addition, some participants may then tend to cling to details, thus consolidating their former, inappropriate perception pattern.

Information Collection

A previously selected picture of low complexity and emotional stress (▶ CD Materials 9) is projected on the screen. The primary therapist directly addresses certain participants, asking them to describe the pictures. If they mostly describe details, these are then summarized. The co-therapist notes down all the resulting information on the flip chart. The primary therapist summarizes this again or lets participants summarize the information themselves. In the case of complex pictures, the primary therapist focuses on different sections of the picture in sequence, e.g., first top left, then in the middle of the picture, or first the background and then the foreground etc. (Fig. 2.17). With this technique, the primary therapist guides the group's attention to relevant target stimuli. The goal is that participants learn to differentiate between relevant and irrelevant stimuli. At the conclusion of this first stage, all the information about the pictures should be noted down on the flip chart. Finally, this information is again summarized in an overview. If participants already offer interpretations and assumptions during information collection, therapists should indeed listen to them. Yet such interpretations are then deferred until the following interpretation and discussion stage.

Example

That is an important point. If I understand it correctly, this is an interpretation. So would it be all right with you if we put your comment aside for now and come back to it? First we want to collect details. The co-therapist has taken a note of your point on the flip chart under the heading of "interpretation".

Interpretation and Discussion

When all the information is collected, the second stage begins: interpretation of the pictures. Therapists should not make interpretations themselves, not even partial

interpretations. Instead, the primary therapist has the following three tasks:
- Encouraging interpretation (possibly by presenting the depicted situation in a role play)
- Supporting interpretation using the facts collected in stage 1
- Encouraging discussion

To encourage interpretation, the primary therapist structures the conversation and focuses on certain picture sections or details as in the information collection stage (e.g., "You said before that the person on the left had a wide-open mouth. What could this mean?"). As a further didactic aid, the therapists could reenact the content of a picture in a role play. Such a use of the therapy materials, which goes beyond the original IPT concept, pursues two aims:
1. **Reducing problems of understanding:** Some participants may find it difficult to understand the images, especially with more complex and emotionally focused pictures. In such cases, active recreation of the depicted scene in a role play helps these participants experience the basic situation actively so they can understand it better. The participant's personal experience of the role play promotes recognition of the essential aspects of a social interaction.
2. **Promoting perspective adoption:** An activating group presentation of picture content requires that the participants involved empathize with the persons depicted in the original image. Participants need to adopt their perspectives. In order to do this, they need to interpret the relationships and feelings of the persons shown on the photographs ("What relationship do the main characters have? How do they feel?") The difference between the objective perception of facts and subjective assumptions is key in this process.

The primary therapist also asks specific questions that force participants to justify their interpretations ("What do you base your claim on that both persons in the picture are excited as they talk to each other? Is there proof of this?"). Finally, the primary therapist encourages discussion of interpretations that have been substantiated ("What do the others have to say about this? Did you arrive at the same conclusion or are there other ways of looking at it?"). Although it is already the interpretation stage, sometimes participants recognize crucial information they did not notice before. Such information is added belatedly to the information list.

As a rule, two or three alternative interpretations of picture details are given. It is advantageous to limit them to three. However, the object is not to convince the participants of a predetermined "correct" interpretation. Instead, the participants should defend their own interpretation with arguments vis-à-vis those of other group members. For example, if two participants can both justify their differing interpretations conclusively, then both interpretation alternatives are accepted as "correct". The therapeutic focus is thus not on "right" or "wrong". Rather, the group should develop the ability to argue logically on the basis of details shown in the image. In this stage, the therapists directly address certain group members to make sure that they do not simply accept the apparently "correct" opinions (interpretations) of others. Rather, each participant should also be able to follow the argument (or assume the perspective of the person making the argument). For this purpose, a participant is directly asked to justify with his or her own words the opinion given by another group member using the information collected in stage 1.

Finding a Title

If stages 1 and 2 have been sufficiently completed, the primary therapist asks each group member to formulate a title or heading for the picture. The title should express the crux of the image concisely. As a rule, the title deals with interpersonal interactions, sometimes with expressions of feeling as well. Original titles (e.g., puns such as are found in advertising) are also accepted as long as they refer to the content of the picture. The titles suggested by the participants are noted on the flip chart and then discussed. As in stage 2, participants are encouraged to defend their titles with arguments and to support their arguments with facts.

Referring the Pictures to the Self and Everyday Life

After the images of both photo series are discussed in the manner described above, participants are encouraged (in contrast to the IPT subprogram "Social Perception") to make connections to themselves and their everyday lives. Every image is compared to equivalent everyday experiences and associated experiences of self-perception.

? Examples of Key Questions
- Have I experienced such situations?
- What feelings and attitudes did I perceive in the other person?
- What did I experience in the process?
- What did I think and feel?
- How was I able to deal with it and how did I react?

Or if participants claim to have had no such experience:
- How would I react in such a situation?

The aim is to associate the therapy/picture content with participants' everyday experiences in order to loosen up habitual perception and reasoning patterns. Again, the distinction between objective facts and assumptions or hypotheses must be observed so as to counteract automatically activated perception patterns. Objective facts and individual hypotheses arising during perception processing are noted down on the flip chart by the co-therapist. The hypotheses are then subjected to a reality check. First the therapist asks the other participants whether they are of the same opinion in the interpretation of the situation or interaction. A group discussion follows. In the process, the therapists assist the participants in putting themselves in the role of the interaction partner ("How would I react? What would I think or feel if I were in that person's shoes? Would I see things the same way as I do now?"). In the case of distorted or inappropriate assumptions (hypotheses), the group finally looks for and discusses alternative hypotheses for processing their perception. However, the discussion should remain focused on the perception of social interactions. The attribution of events is discussed in Module D.

Adopting the Perspective of Others

The subject of perspective adoption (ToM) was already introduced using the two picture series (▶ CD Materials 9a–g). This will now be explored further. In doing this, the therapist first returns to the techniques of emotional perception learned in Module A (▶ CD Information Sheets 7 and 8). This is done remind the group that appropriate affect decoding is one of the requirements for perspective adoption.

Example of an Introductory Exercise

As agreed with the primary therapist during session preparation, the co-therapist suddenly cries out, hits himself or herself on the cheek (as if stung by a mosquito), and then swears angrily. Immediately, the primary therapist asks the group: "Does anyone know what happened?" The participants usually recognize instantly what might have happened to the co-therapist. The objective of the group discussion is to find out why the participants came to this correct conclusion. How did you orient yourself? What facts did you make use of? Was it your own experience with mosquito bites and the resultant emotional expression (crying out, anger), bodily sensation (pain), consequential actions (striking or chasing away the mosquito), and verbal utterances ("Damned mosquito!")?

In addition, ▶ CD Information Sheet 18 ("Empathizing with others") on the enclosed ▶ CD-ROM is now distributed and read. The distinction between (objective) facts and (hypothetical) assumptions is reiterated. The objective is to list facts we might use in adopting another person's perspective in the light of our own experience. The following is an example of such a list.

a. Social rules (e.g., "Everybody does that", game rules)
b. Nonverbal
   - Emotional expressions of others (e.g., facial expressions, gestures)
   - Typical behavior (e.g., movement patterns, eye contact)
c. Verbal
   - Spoken or written content
   - Tone and speed when speaking
d. Situational conditions (e.g., place, surroundings, other people present)

Social rules serve here only as orientation aids for perspective adoption. Rule violations will be discussed later in Module C (social schemas). All facts are listed on the flip chart as orientation aids for perspective adoption. The therapist also addresses techniques that make it easier to adopt the perspective of another person. One possible key question in this context is:

? What helps me in my everyday life to adopt the perspective of others – to put myself in their shoes?

Participants' comments are once again recorded on the flip chart. These are supplemented by ▶ CD Information Sheet 18 ("Empathizing with others"), which was read earlier, and ▶ CD Information Sheet 19 ("Possible ways to help increase our empathy with others"). On the latter, participants note additional means of assistance that were not included and may have been mentioned previously in group discussion.

In conformity with usual INT didactic method, this is now followed by practical group exercises so the participants can try out the techniques (means of assistance) of perspective adoption for the first time. Three exercises will be presented in the following:

- Water, reflections, mountains, old city, birds (▶ CD e-Materials 6a–e)
- Sentences on perspective adoption (▶ CD Materials 10a–c)
- Film excerpts

Landscapes, Cities, and People The group is split up into two teams. One team leaves the room for a few minutes along with the co-therapist. During this time, this team performs simple exercises (e.g., memory exercises using ▶ CD Materials 9) or has a break. In the meantime, the primary therapist shows the team remaining in the group room a single picture (target picture) via digital projector from the picture series of ▶ CD e-Materials 6a–e. The task of this team is to describe the picture as concisely and in as much detail as possible. They should also consider which of the picture's (essential) features could help the other team recognize the picture. Their contributions are taken down on the flip chart. One or two members of this team must now remember all the picture descriptions made by the team (notes are permitted) so they can present them

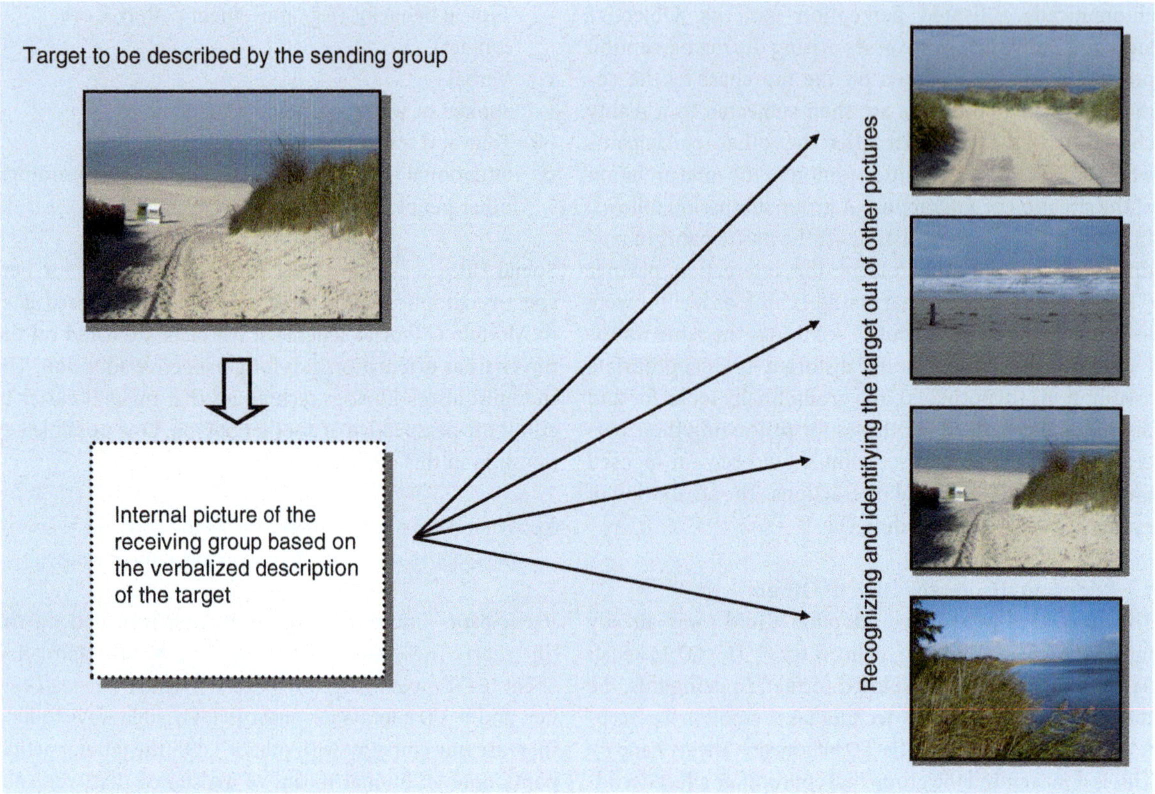

Fig. 2.18 Perspective adoption: exercise "landscapes and cities" (Photos: F. Perret and S. Schmidt, with kind permission)

later to the other team. This presentation is practiced briefly and supplemented or corrected by other team members if required. In this way, this group has now become the "transmitter group" of information about the target picture. When they are finished practicing transmitting/presenting, the primary therapist removes the projected image and asks the second team with the co-therapist into the group room. The latter team now becomes the receiver group and hears a verbal description of the target picture without seeing it. The receiver group is instructed to make as good a mental image of the described picture as possible (internal picture) and to describe the picture with their own words. Then the entire picture series, some of whose pictures are similar to the target picture, is shown (▶ CD e-Materials 6a or 6b). Each time a picture is shown, the "receiver group" discusses whether the current one corresponds to the target picture. The team should give reasons why a picture does not correspond to the target picture. Errors of omission or confusion are discussed, as well as deviations from one's own memory in case of correctly recognized images. If the target picture has been identified, the teams exchange their previously assigned roles. The exercise's level of difficulty can be varied by the selection of target picture (the more similar the target picture is with one or more of the other pictures, the more difficult it is to identify it). The difficulty level can also be altered by changing the picture's position within the series (the later the target picture is shown in the series, the larger the probability of false conclusions). Fig. 2.18 is a diagram of this exercise.

Sentences on Perspective Adoption Sentences on perspective adoption are printed on cards, one or two per card. These sentences concisely describe a situation in which a person is experiencing something (▶ CD Materials 10a–c). Examples of such cards labeled with sentences are shown in Fig. 2.19. These cards are designed for two potential uses:

1. One participant receives a card and reads the text on it to the group. The group then discusses the associated feeling ("What does this person think and feel during this experience?"). This situation is also referred to patients' self-perception and everyday lives ("What would I think and feel? How would I react if that were to happen to me in my everyday life?").
2. On a higher difficulty level, the situations described on the cards are performed in a role play. Two variations are possible:

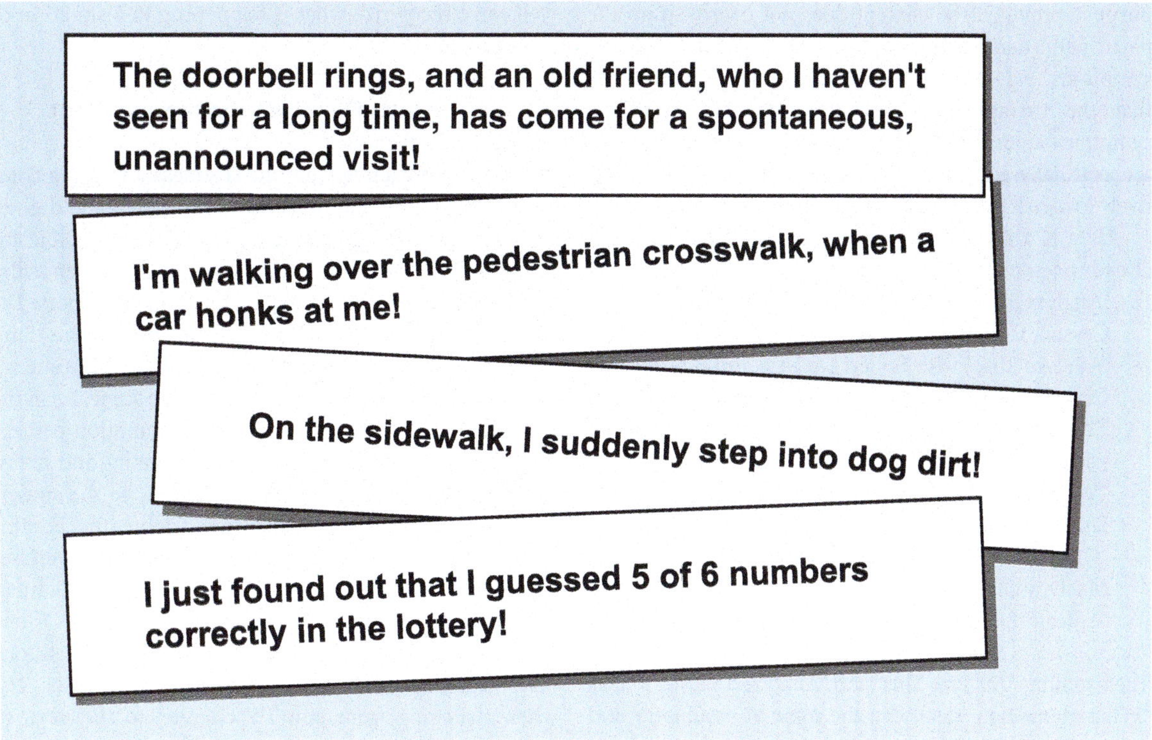

Fig. 2.19 Perspective adoption: exercise "sentences on perspective adoption"

a. One participant receives a card and performs the described situation. The other group members then try to place themselves in this situation. They try to recognize which features of the situation the first participant was acting out, what feeling he or she expressed, and what he or she was thinking at the time.
b. Some cards are also suitable for group exercises in which an unprepared patient has direct, realistic experiences. This will now be explained using the card with the sentence "Just as I'm walking across the crosswalk, a car honks!" as an example:

Example

One participant is asked to leave the group room accompanied by the co-therapist. This participant has not been instructed of what he or she should expect on returning. The rest of the group is introduced to the role play on the card. The therapist instructs the participants to imagine they are each sitting in the car of their choice, which is stopped in a queue in front of a crosswalk. Usually luxury cars or sports cars are chosen. After this, the participants find out that some of the pedestrians are taking an extremely long time to use the crosswalk. This is annoying the drivers, all of whom are under a lot of time pressure. All the drivers are in a hurry. If the target patient (together with the co-therapist) now walks along the imaginary crosswalk particularly slowly, they are then to honk their horns as loudly as possible. Precisely this takes place. The target patient returns and is instructed exclusively by the co-therapist to walk slowly across the imaginary crosswalk. At the conclusion of this (usually highly activating) exercise, both the target patient and the "honking drivers" are asked how they felt, what they thought, and how they would react in everyday life if they heard honking on the crosswalk or had to wait a long time in the car in front of the crosswalk while in a hurry.

Film Excerpts A film scene is played for the participants using the projector. The therapist then gives them the following tasks:
1. To give a detailed description of the scene
2. To describe the characters using concrete facts from the film
3. To interpret the plot or interactions between characters using facts from the film
4. To place themselves within the scene that was shown and to try to feel out what was happening in the film prior to it. What led to the scene that was shown?
5. To connect the scene with the participants' everyday lives: How would I have reacted in this scene? Have I had such experiences in my everyday life?

Commercially available DVDs can be drawn upon for film material. In principle, most films are suitable for the purpose provided the content does not overly strain the participants and does not interfere with existing delusion symptoms (e.g., secret agent or cop films). This requires that the therapists are aware of possible persisting symptoms among all the participants. As a rule, comedies are especially good for this purpose since they are relatively low-risk but still activate the viewers.

Here is a selection of recommended films that have already been used:

- "Analyze This", with Robert De Niro and Billy Crystal, USA 1999
- "Analyze That", with Robert De Niro and Billy Crystal, USA 2002
- "There's Something About Mary", with Cameron Diaz and Ben Stiller, USA 1998
- "What About Bob?", with Bill Murray and Richard Dreifuss, USA 1991
- "Groundhog Day", with Bill Murray and Andie MacDowell, USA 1993
- "A Beautiful Mind", with Russell Crowe, USA 2001

The two films "Analyze This" and "Analyze That" as well as "What about Bob" deal with the topic of psychiatry and psychotherapy. This theme is also explored in "A Beautiful Mind". However, only predominately comedic scenes are recommended. For scene selection, the DVD scene menu can be used, because these are usually self-contained sections of the film. The level of difficulty of the scenes depends on plot complexity, emotional stress, and the position of the scene within the overall plot of the film (the earlier the scene, the less information is lacking about plot).

2.3.2.2.3 Restitution

In the restitution section, newly learned strategies for affect decoding are now practiced to the point of habituation. In this module section, no additional exercises are available. Instead, therapists should use the exercises in the compensation section. The two photo series on social perception (▶ CD Materials 9a–g) and the photo series on perspective adoption (▶ CD e-Materials 6) as well as the exercises "Sentences on perspective adoption" (▶ CD Materials 10a–c) and "Film excerpts" give the participants ample material for repeated practice and learning in the group. The difficulty level of the exercises can now be gradually increased following the procedure described above. Referring back to ▶ CD Information Sheets 16–19, each participant fills in ▶ CD Worksheet 4 ("My helpful strategies for …") again individually before every exercise unit. At the end of this intervention section, participants add to or correct their initial self-assessments with respect to social perception and perspective adoption skills on ▶ CD Worksheet 11 ("How well can I recognize what is happening in a situation or a conversation?").

2.3.2.2.4 In Vivo Exercises and Independent Exercises

As an in vivo exercise that fits seamlessly into the compensation and restitution section, the group could go to the cinema together. If a group visit is impossible for organizational reasons, participants can also watch a film of their choice in pairs or with a few group members. The film is then discussed following the formula of the "Film excerpts" exercise. The difference is that this time an entire film is being absorbed, not just one scene. As in the previous social-cognitive target area of emotion perception, this in vivo exercise may be too activating and stressful for the participants. Many avoid going to the cinema because they consider it stressful and frightening. For this reason, it is sometimes preferable to configure exercises on social perception and perspective adoption in a more passive way, from the perspective of an observer. Or one can refer to more familiar surroundings. In this case, one possible independent exercise could be as follows: Try, when switching from one TV channel to the next, to remain focused on a program or film that has already begun and to find out what is happening. Another independent exercise is to observe other people at a restaurant, a park, at work or even one's own domestic environment to find out what and how these people are communicating (verbal and nonverbal content). ▶ CD Worksheet 5 ("Independent exercise") is filled out to prepare for each independent or in vivo exercise. Subsequent discussion follows the procedure described in the previous intervention unit.

2.3.3 INT Module C

Module C primarily addresses the neurocognitive target area of the executive functions, particularly reasoning and problem solving. Reasoning encompasses cognitive flexibility and concept formation. The concept of problem solving also incorporates planning skills. As before, coping skills acquired in previous modules are required for successful interventions in this area. Some group members may still exhibit considerable limitations in the basal cognitive functions previously described and may have insufficiently appropriated the coping strategies discussed. If so, some of the steps from Modules A and B should be repeated before starting Module C.

The social-cognitive section of Module C contains interventions for the target area of social schemas, also called social knowledge. These are automatic patterns of thought and behavior derived from social roles and rules (norms). Moreover, social schemas can lie behind prejudices such as the stigma of psychiatric illness. This intervention topic is usually identified with emotional strain. All participants have had negative experiences of violating social roles and rules as well as the consequences of this. Therefore, the intervention initially makes didactic use of scripts with less emotional impact. Finally, after gradually increasing the degree of emotional strain, the group discusses coping with the stigma of illness.

2.3.3.1 Neurocognitive Intervention Area: Reasoning and Problem Solving

Module C: Neurocognitive Intervention Area: Reasoning and Problem Solving

1. Introduction: reasoning and problem solving
   - Definition: cognitive flexibility and concept formation
   - Semantic network model
   - Goal orientation
   - Self-perception in the target area (cognitive profile)
   - Reference to everyday life and self: case vignette
2. Compensation
   - Learning and individualizing coping strategies:
     - Goal orientation and definition
     - Obstacles in realizing goals
     - Goal realization in 6 steps
     - Realizing individual goals in everyday life
     - Planning action
     - Concept formation: finding the right words
3. Restitution
   - Habituation of learned coping strategies:
     - Repetition of group exercises
     - Computer exercises
4. In vivo exercises and independent exercises
   - Transfer of individualized coping strategies to concrete, everyday situations

Tips

- Infrastructure: group therapy and computer rooms, flip chart, digital projector
- Therapy materials: ► CD Information Sheets 3–15, 20–26, ► CD Worksheets 4, 12–15, ► CD Vignettes 11–12, ► CD Materials 1–2, 5, 11–13
- CogPack exercises: SCALES, LABYRINTHS, ANAGRAMS, GUESSWORDS, CONCEPTS, CONFUSION
- Didactics: structured group discussion, group exercises, computer exercises (individual and group)

2.3.3.1.1 Introductory Sessions

■ Reasoning

■■ Definition of the Target Area: Reasoning

The faculty of reasoning is the object of various scientific disciplines. INT focuses on the neurocognitive function of reasoning, which is generally measured by the capacity to form (verbal) concepts and cognitive flexibility. In INT, this function is psychotherapeutically operationalized. Concept formation is the ability to categorize and distinguish different linguistic and emotional stimuli or symbols. Cognitive flexibility is the ability to apply acquired knowledge flexibly and appropriately to the situation.

Reasoning processes (concept formation and cognitive flexibility) are also necessary when solving concrete problems and planning. This module deals with both of these neurocognitive functions, reasoning and problem solving. The definition of terms starts with the function of reasoning.

The concept of reasoning or thinking is used often in everyday language. Also, patients suffering from schizophrenia often use the term to subjectively describe illness-related symptoms ("I can't think clearly anymore", "My thoughts are going in circles again"). In light of this, two possible ways of establishing a uniform definition present themselves:

- Group discussion: Starting with the key question: "What does the term 'thinking' mean for you?", the group defines the concept under the guidance of the primary therapist using everyday examples. The contributions of the participants should be summarized and categorized on the flip chart by the co-therapist. This somewhat time-intensive method can be highly activating and motivating for the participants. The difficulty is in keeping the discussion focused exclusively on neurocognitive aspects of reasoning.
- The primary therapist introduces the topic while referring back to the cognitive topics of Modules A and B.

Introduction Example

We will now turn our attention to our faculties of thinking or reasoning. You could say that everybody thinks. But what does this mean? We all use this term differently in our everyday lives. Some say: "When we think, we're active. So we become tired if we think too much". Others say: "Thinking requires knowledge! If you don't know much about a certain subject, you can't think about it very well" or "Thinking is logical, but sometimes we think spontaneously and automatically, which isn't always logical". Still others say: "Thought is the knowledge we obtain from our own ideas and experiences" and "Thinking takes place in the brain". These propositions are of course all correct. But what is important for us is this: Thinking takes place above all using concepts. Thinking, or reasoning, is thus the flexible application of what we have learned from our life experiences. Yet reasoning also means associating new information with stored information.

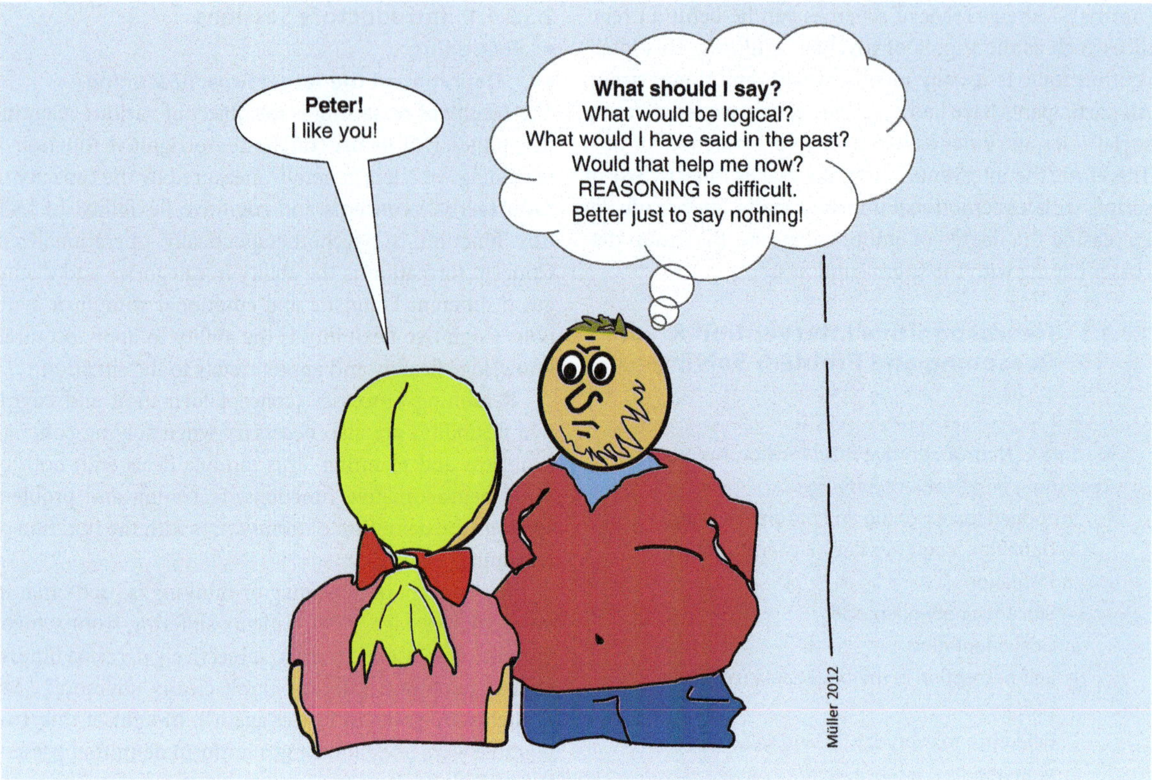
Peter!
I like you!
What should I say?
What would be logical?
What would I have said in the past?
Would that help me now?
REASONING is difficult.
Better just to say nothing!
Müller 2012

Fig. 2.20 Information sheet: flexible use of language and concept formation in an emotionally stressful interaction

The therapist refers back to previously discussed cognitive topics and introduces relevant models of (verbal) concept formation and cognitive flexibility. ► CD Information Sheet 20 ("I think, therefore I am") is available on the ► CD-ROM for this purpose. The information sheet talks about using words flexibly in an emotionally stressful interaction (Fig. 2.20). After reading the information sheet, group discussion relates the topic to the participants' everyday experiences.

Examples of Key Questions

- How would you react in this situation? Would you have found the right words?
- Have you already had comparable experiences? What did you do then?

Semantic Network Model

Now that concept formation has been introduced, it is now illustrated with the help of neural networks. For this, semantic network models are used. Therapists should avoid specialized neurological and medical terminology. Instead, they should explain simply why it is sometimes difficult to find the right words in a conversation or during a thought process. ► CD Information Sheet 21 ("Reasoning, a matter of the brain") is available for this purpose. Semantic network models (reasoning and cognitive flexibility) provide the theoretical framework for understanding the retrieval and use of information stored in memory. According to these models, memory content is arranged as a network in the brain in the form of neural nodes. Stored information (representations, concepts) is accessed by activating these nodes. The objective is to improve participants' arrangement of semantic information (concept formation, category formation).

After the participants read ► CD Information Sheet 21, the following group exercise illustrates the semantic network model:

Assigning Concepts The primary therapist mentions a term (e.g., car, milk, dancing, etc.). The participants are asked to name any words or concepts that occur to them. These are noted on the flip chart and connected to each other using a method analogous to the example on ► CD Information Sheet 21. Concepts that are directly related to the initial term (e.g., car) are written down and connected spatially closer to that term (e.g., wheels, steering wheel, vehicle). Concepts that are only vaguely associated (usually via a subordinate term) are written farther away (e.g., bicycles also have wheels and are also means of transport). This then results in a structure composed of concepts on several levels, in the center of which is the initial term. After naming the main concept (car), the participants name the concepts of the first level of association (wheels, steering wheel, vehicle), followed by those of the second and third level of association (bicycle). This exercise serves to demonstrate the activation of neural nodes during the thought process.

▪▪ Promoting Self-Perception in the Cognitive Target Area

Therapists refer the topic to patients' self-perception and everyday experiences using the same didactic means as were described already in Module A and B. Participants are first asked how they assess their own reasoning skills. They are also asked, if possible, to describe a concrete situation or report an event from their everyday lives. Participants' statements regarding concrete situations are recorded on the flip chart. In addition, each participant fills out ▶ CD Worksheet 12 ("How well can I reason in my everyday life?").

▪▪ Case Vignettes

The group now reads ▶ CD Vignette 11 ("One film – two summaries") paragraph by paragraph. After reading the vignette, group discussion relates the vignette to the participants' own experiences. Discussion should center on the social aspect of reasoning and its importance in communication. Since the vignette contains two very different attempts to summarize the same film, the participants are first asked with which description they can identify (or which they clearly disagree with). Concrete life experiences with the topic are summarized. Therapists should always stress participant resources when discussing the reasoning functions. Possible key questions for promoting self-reflection include:

? Examples of Key Questions

- Have there been situations when I had to find the right words to tell a story from my own life so that others could relate to it?
- Has this happened often?
- In which situations did that go well? When did I have problems?

Also the following general questions for self-reflection:

- Is it easy for me to relate something to others? Do I usually find the words?
- Am I the kind of person who usually says little and has problems expressing himself/herself?
- Are there moments when I have the feeling that people don't understand me?
- Are my thoughts sometimes very rapid and imaginative? Do I have so many ideas that it's difficult to express the most crucial things so that people can understand me?

The group now explores individual, subjective experiences of strengths and weaknesses in reasoning using everyday life situations. Again, any coping strategies participants volunteer at this time are noted for subsequent discussion in the compensation section.

▪ Problem Solving

At this point, the second neurocognitive target area of problem solving is introduced. This is understood as a further aspect or function of reasoning. Accordingly, the compensation section will deal simultaneously with coping strategies for both functions: reasoning and problem solving.

▪▪ Definition of the Target Area: Problem Solving

The focus of this definition is on the planning, preparation, and execution of actions in order to realize goals. This is contrasted with spontaneous approaches to solving problems that lack a clear plan of action (trial – error). The didactic focus is thus aimed at developing solution strategies and subdividing problem solving processes into separate solution steps. The overriding objective is to sensitize participants for goal/solution-oriented thinking and behavior in everyday life. In this way, they will better be able to plan and reach individual goals and meet their own needs.

Introduction Example

The reasoning functions we have already discussed are also necessary when we try to solve a problem in our everyday lives. Now how do we define a problem and its solution? To put it somewhat abstractly, a problem consists in the discrepancy between the existing ACTUAL state and the desired TARGET state. Overcoming this discrepancy or arriving at the TARGET state is the solution of the problem. For example, say that our shoes are worn out (ACTUAL state). We then need a new pair of shoes (TARGET state). The problem is then defined by the question of how we are to obtain new shoes and what we have to factor in to obtain them. In order to solve this problem, we are faced with two possibilities:

- We could try to solve the problem spontaneously by trial and error. That is, we could buy shoes somewhere and somehow without giving it any prior thought. The disadvantage of this is that we have no guarantee of obtaining new shoes within a short time.
- So we plan the action by setting a concrete goal (e.g., black, lined winter shoes, which shouldn't be too expensive). We take potential difficulties into account (I need a driver's license to get to town, only have free time the day after tomorrow etc.). We also develop different alternative strategies for when, how, and where we can get new shoes (I'm going to one of the footwear discounters I known in town on the weekend with my sister or a friend).

As before, it is recommended that the therapist point out patients' personal resources and difficulties in problem solving, since the ensuing compensation section will build upon participant resources to a great extent. In addition, therapists should distinguish between solution possibilities that lend themselves to planning and more immediate problems that require a spontaneous solution.

▪▪ Promoting Self-Perception in the Cognitive Target Area

Again, asking participants how they usually assess their own problem solving skills helps relate the topic to their everyday experiences. Participants' statements regarding concrete situations are recorded on the flip chart. In addition, each participant fills out ► CD Worksheet 13 ("How well can I solve problems?").

▪▪ Case Vignettes

► CD Vignette 12 ("Planning the trip to the cinema") is used as a didactic tool to elicit participants' resources/strengths and weaknesses. The story of the protagonist Peter is read paragraph-by-paragraph in the group and then discussed. This is followed by specific questions in order to promote reflection about everyday life:

? Examples of Key Questions

- What do I do when I want to go to the cinema? Do I rely on other people to plan the trip and pick out the film? What is my contribution in the process, or what prevents me from going to the cinema?
- Is it easy for me to decide on something, to be active? What hinders me from this?
- Do I identify my everyday problems and try to solve them or do I often tend to sweep problems under the carpet so I won't have to think of them? Why is that the case?

Then the group discusses and categorizes subjectively experienced strengths and weaknesses involved in solving problems. Any coping strategies mentioned in the process are recorded on the flip chart for later use in the compensation section.

▪▪ Factors Influencing Reasoning and Problem Solving

On the basis of the group's concrete, everyday experiences, factors that might impede situation-appropriate reasoning and problem solving are now discussed. If too few or too specific everyday situations have been described by the participants, one of the following topics can also be addressed:

- **Active organization of leisure time:** hobbies, activities, daily structure, interests, etc.
- **Work situation:** cooperation with coworkers, amusement during breaks, instructions from the boss, work time, conflicts, etc.
- **Living situation:** interaction with roommates and neighbors, housekeeping, shopping, etc.
- **Relationships:** establishing contacts, conversing with coworkers, asserting oneself, expressing interpersonal feelings, etc.

The goal is to sensitize participants to factors that may affect reasoning. ► CD Information Sheet 22 ("What affects our ability to reason and solve problems?") is available for this purpose on the enclosed ► CD-ROM. This describes influences on the functions of reasoning and problem solving made by acute emotional strain, mood, and stress. It also describes the effects of the previously discussed neurocognitive functions, speed of information processing, attention, and memory. Accordingly, a further function of ► CD Information Sheet 22 is to review Modules A and B, presenting the participants with a recurrent theme running through the INT group process. Further everyday influences on the functions of reasoning and problem solving experienced by the participants can be added to the information sheet. These influential factors, once analyzed and compiled, function as a basis for the following compensation section. One exception is the experience of stress, coping strategies for which will first be dealt with in the Module D.

2.3.3.1.2 Compensation

The compensation section combines coping strategies for both neurocognitive functions, reasoning and problem solving. Problem solving is defined as reasoning applied to planning and concrete sequences of action. First, goal-oriented reasoning and action are introduced. This serves as the prerequisite for problem solving. The group then discusses problems finding the correct words in a social context. This difficulty in interpersonal interactions also serves as a link to the following social-cognitive section on social schemas.

▪ Goal Orientation

The group first requires a didactic conceptual clarification of the intervention objective: goal realization versus problem solving. Solving a problem is reformulated accordingly as reaching a previously defined goal. The aim is to establish goal-oriented action and reasoning among the participants. For the purpose of illustration and of facilitating concrete experience, the following group exercise (► CD Materials 11) can be carried out:

A Group Matchstick Exercise The primary therapist has brought a box of matchsticks or toothpicks. He places

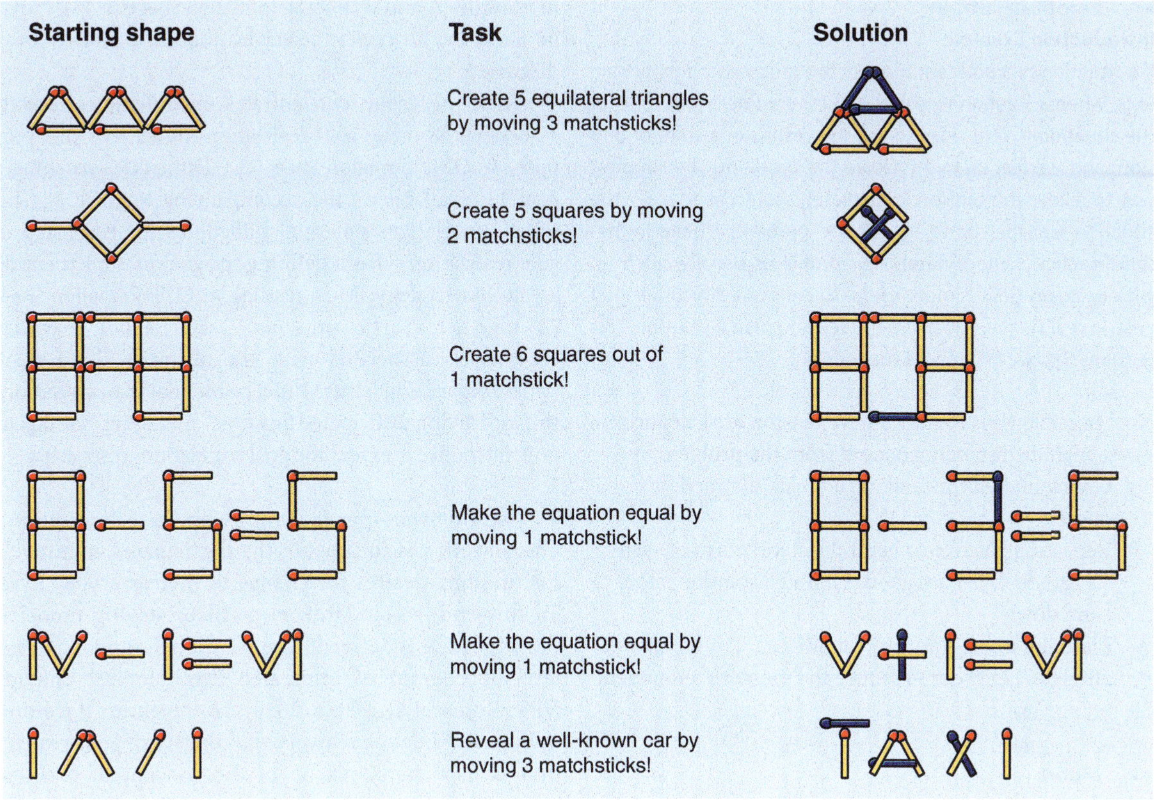

Fig. 2.21 Group matchstick exercise

them beside one of the original figures or equations shown in Fig. 2.21 and then assigns the task written beside it. (The solutions are on the right). The group now attempts to solve the problem spontaneously. The primary therapist structures group discussion such that they first define the goal (what should the figure or equation look like?), summarize the means/rules available to achieve this (how many matchsticks may be moved?) and possible strategies (which matchsticks are more suitable and why?). Finally, they decide upon one of these strategies as a group in a consensus-oriented way. After one or two tasks have been solved, the primary therapist asks the group what helped and what hindered solving the problem. Could they develop strategies? The therapist also asks whether everyone in the group had a say and what would have been different if the task had been solved alone instead of as a group.

Obstacles in Realizing Goals

Participants may have already volunteered obstacles and difficulties in realizing goals in the introductory section as well as in the previous exercise. These are now compiled. In addition, the primary therapist refers back to self-assessments of functionality in the various cognitive domains, especially in the areas of reasoning and problem solving (▶ CD Worksheets 12 and 13). Combined, these make up the individual cognitive profile of each participant. They contain both weaknesses and strengths. Of course, the person concerned can exhibit a partial weakness in the cognitive function of reasoning and problem solving – just as there might be strengths in other cognitive functions. The primary therapist summarizes weaknesses described by participants in thinking and problem solving accordingly. Moreover, it is helpful and relieving for most participants when the primary therapist points out time and again that he or she has never met someone whose cognitive profile consists exclusively of cognitive strengths. The goal is to encourage such participants, despite weaknesses in the target area, to engage themselves with the exercises and to improve their own functional abilities by trying out new coping strategies.

The influential factors listed on ▶ CD Information Sheet 22 ("What affects our ability to reason and solve problems?") and others that may have been added are now discussed as possible obstacles to goal-realization. Therapists should also address possible coping strategies for reducing negative influences.

2

Emotional Strain

Introduction Example

If a situation or a problem triggers too much emotional strain (e.g., when a solution to a problem is very important to us or the situation is very close to us), this results in a state of tension, and we feel unable to solve the problem. The simplest way to relieve this tension immediately would be to leave the situation (escape) or to ignore the problem ("head-in-the-sand" tactics). Unfortunately, our problems usually catch up with us again. So it is more useful to confront difficulties that arise in realizing our goal and to seek and plan a solution. This requires that we first relieve the tension.

Now possible ways to help relieve tension are categorized. These include distancing oneself from the problem by

- Giving oneself time, taking a break, distracting oneself
- Repeating positive or neutral statements to oneself ("I can do this, I am good, I'll find a solution, etc.") to calm down
- Planning to ask someone for advice ("I'm not alone after all!") in order to reduce the pressure on oneself.

Mood

Introduction Example

Sometimes we simply don't feel like racking our brains about a problem. Usually we opt for one of two possibilities: Either we postpone tackling the problem until later in the hope that it will be easier then, or we try to motivate ourselves and confront the problem.

And:

The option of "postponing till later" involves the risk of delaying confronting our problems too long. Often the only way out of this dilemma is to keep fixed deadlines, similar to homework assignments in school.

Or:

How do we motivate ourselves? It often helps to reinforce ourselves when we reward ourselves with something. Is also helps when we consider the fact that, when we have finished something, often a great weight is dropped from our shoulders. This is a good feeling!

The Experience of Stress

Dealing with stress is first dealt with in Module D. Associated coping experiences and suggestions offered by the participants are noted on the flip chart, but they are set aside for now to be reintroduced in Module D.

Concentration and Memory Problems

If basal cognitive deficits that interfere with executive functioning exist, therapists can refer back to the coping strategies for improving these functions already handled in Modules A and B (▶ CD Information Sheets 3–15). It may be necessary to review strategies that have already been discussed.

Then the group concentrates on difficulties directly associated with the goal realization model. For this purpose, ▶ CD Information Sheet 23 ("Difficulties reaching a goal") is available on the accompanying ▶ CD-ROM. This sheet summarizes potential difficulties for each step of goal realization – from defining the goal to implementing a solution strategy. After reading ▶ CD Information Sheet 23 together, participants are asked about everyday experiences associated with the obstacles listed there (work, organizing leisure time, residential issues, relationships). Having anticipated possible difficulties, therapists now introduce a model for goal realization in six steps.

Coping Strategies for Improving Goal-Realization

The objective is to prepare the participants cognitively for fulfilling desires for change in their everyday lives. To this end, a standardized problem solving model is introduced. It is derived from the model provided in the last subprogram of Integrated Psychological Therapy (IPT; Roder et al. 2008a, 2010). However, for the aforementioned didactic reasons, the concept of goal-realization is used here instead of the concept of problem solving.

The process of goal-realization is subdivided into six steps:

1. Defining the goal
2. Alternative ways to realize the goal
3. Evaluating these alternatives and their consequences
4. Deciding on one of these alternatives
5. Planning and implementing
6. Reviewing the success of the action

These six steps of goal-realization are summarized on ▶ CD Information Sheet 24 ("Steps for reaching a goal") of the enclosed ▶ CD-ROM and will be described in the following:

1. Goal Definition

The first step of the intervention is defining the problem. First, assumptions have to be distinguished from facts. If necessary, idiosyncratic perspectives must be corrected. Complex problems should be broken down into smaller problems. The objective is to encourage a pragmatic and change-oriented attitude and to work out concrete and realistic personal goals. In the case of patients with schizophrenia, one should expect experience-related and illness-related resistance. Perception based on assumptions and beliefs – also applied to real problems – sometimes impedes access to one's own needs. This makes it very difficult to realize personal goals. Many schizophrenia patients associate changes with great strain, which often preempts attempts to change. For this reason, insight into personal problems should be promoted at the start of the goal-realization intervention. Participants should be encouraged to be open to change and supported in defining realistic goals. Pointing out the positive aspects of goal-realization usually helps ("How would you feel if you had reached that goal?"). The following example from an actual INT session can serves as a model for each step of the goal-realization process:

Example

At the start, the therapist describes a problem from his own everyday life. He would like to go to a match of the European Football Championship, which will be taking place in his hometown among other places. The problem is that he is having difficulty leaving his family alone again. Moreover, the tickets for the good games are already sold out. The group chooses a subproblem: getting an admission ticket.

▪▪ 2. Alternatives for Realizing the Goal

When the individual goal has been defined, the second step is to find possible ways to realize the goal. Cognitive flexibility is addressed here in the form of brainstorming in order to obtain as many different alternatives as possible. However, the alternatives should not be evaluated yet. This also means that the therapists should positively reinforce all the alternatives suggested. Initially, alternatives are collected in the context of the entire group. Later the participants should acquire the skill of generating various goal-realization alternatives independently.

Example (Continued)

In a brainstorming session, the following goal-realization alternatives are generated:

a. The therapist hypnotizes the ticket inspector at the football stadium.
b. The therapist tells the ticket inspector that he has to get into the stadium with a psychiatric patient for therapeutic reasons.
c. The therapist climbs into the stadium through the toilet window illegally.
d. The therapist purchases an (overpriced) scalped ticket just before the game.
e. The therapist tries to get a ticket on the Internet.

▪▪ 3. Evaluating the Goal-Realization Alternatives and Their Consequences

Only after all the different alternatives for goal-realization have been compiled does the group begin to assess each alternative and its consequences. This assessment should – as has already been mentioned – not only take into account one's own wants and needs. It should also take into account how rational and realizable the alternative is. Considering the consequences of an action helps the participants in evaluating alternative ways of behaving realistically and in anticipating expected difficulties. Finally, each alternative way to realize the goal is assessed separately. The focus is on the personal benefit of the person concerned. A standard number scale of 1–10 or 1–100 is recommended.

Example (Continued)

The therapist evaluates all the alternatives noted on the flip chart by assigning points (scale of 1–10: 10="I can definitely imagine doing that").

▪▪ 4. Deciding on One of These Alternatives

The decision in favor of one alternative is based on the rational individual assessment of the previous step. The final decision is made solely by the person concerned. The primary therapist can try to intervene correctively and point out an alternative's feasibility, potential difficulties, or probability of success.

Example (Continued)

Only alternative e "The therapist tries to get a ticket on the Internet" receives 10 points from the therapist and is thus selected by him.

▪▪ 5. Planning and Implementing

If a particular course of action for realizing the goal has been determined, the next step is practical implementation. This step is subdivided into two parts. Prior to implementation, a detailed plan is made. If the selected courses of action or behavior patterns are complex, then they are broken down into separate steps and put in sequence. Expected difficulties are now put in concrete terms for each of the action steps.

Example (Continued)

The attempt to acquire a ticket on the Internet was subdivided into the following steps:

1. Ask someone how and where tickets are offered on the Internet.
2. Determine a maximum amount of money (how much might it cost?)
3. Supply and demand: when will it be the most affordable?
4. Make a bid
5. Ask when and where the ticket will be delivered
6. Go to the football game

▪▪ 6. Reviewing the Success of the Action

If a particular course of action has been tried out, a feedback session takes place. Participants have the opportunity to report about their experiences. It is important that every approach is reinforced with concrete coping strategies and target behavior. Poor outcomes and aborted actions are interpreted not as failures but as incentives for correcting the target behavior. This means that the participant concerned is accompanied back to step three ("3. Evaluating the goal-realization alternatives and their consequences"). If necessary, the assessments are adjusted or another alternative is selected, which is now classified as more promising.

Example (Continued)
The therapist tells the group about his difficult acquisition of the ticket and finally about his visit to the football stadium.

Two very different exercises are available at this point. Both give the participants a chance to have their first experiences in applying the goal-realization model. The first is a group exercise with cubes for abstract problem solving. The second is an individual exercise for goal-realization in everyday life.

Cube Exercise The template of a color cube is available on the accompanying ▶ CD-ROM (▶ CD Materials 12a). This should be printed out a total of nine times. The nine templates can then easily be folded together and glued at the given folds to make three-dimensional cubes. The task is formulated on the next materials sheet (▶ CD Materials 12b). The group has to place four or nine cubes (depending on the pattern) on a predefined pattern. The pattern templates should also be printed out beforehand (▶ CD Materials 12c: Sheets 12.1–12.20). The pattern templates increase gradually in difficulty. Pattern sheets 12.1–12.10 require placing four cubes, while the last sheets 12.9–12.10 each contain a pattern, which cannot be reproduced with the cubes. The objective is that the participants (a) recognize that the pattern cannot be placed and (b) that they argue why this is so. The pattern templates 12.11–12.20 require nine cubes. The last two pattern templates (12.19–12.20) contain patterns that can only be solved three-dimensionally. That is, two cubes (12.19) or one cube (12.20) have to be placed on top of the other seven/eight cubes so that the pattern template is recognizable from an aerial perspective. At this point, the group should do no more than two or three patterns. The exercise is repeated later in the restitution section. The therapists should involve all the participants in the solution process by addressing them specifically. Many solution strategies (alternatives ways of realizing the goal) should be worked out in the group (e.g., starting with the corners of the template, subdividing the template by imagination into cube squares, etc.). This exercise can be done as a competition: one half of the group counts the seconds out loud needed by the other half to solve the task as a team.

Individual Goal-Realization in Everyday Life This intervention is concerned with implementing the goal-realization model by means of an individually experienced problem. The objective is that each participant names at least one individual everyday problem and, from this, derives a personal goal. Aside from the practical implementation, goal-processing and feedback sessions take place as a group. This intervention generally requires several sessions. Often only one or two problems can be processed per session. Practical implementation is carried out between the sessions. The following session then starts with a feedback round before the problems of other participants are discussed. As an orientation aid, participants receive ▶ CD Worksheet 14 ("My personal goal") from the ▶ CD-ROM for each implementation. The biggest difficulty in this exercise is finding realistic goals in the initial phase. It is thus the job of the therapists to guide the participants towards clearly structured, quickly realizable goals. Some real examples include: improving social contacts, asserting one's rights, trying out a new recreational activity, getting back a driver's license.

▪ Planning Action

Some participants often experience difficulties planning a course of action and subdividing this into separate steps. Accordingly, cognitive flexibility in planning concrete action steps is discussed in addition to the model of goal-realization. The foremost goal is to use concrete examples from participants' everyday lives to generate action steps and then to order these in a goal-oriented sequence. As opposed to the more complex social action goals of the subsequent exercise in the social-cognitive area on social schemas, the examples here are limited to the purely cognitive domain. To help orient the participants, ▶ CD Information Sheet 25 ("From a complicated action to small action steps") is available on the enclosed ▶ CD-ROM. The following group exercise can provide the participants with their first experiences with goal-oriented action planning in partial steps:

On the ▶ CD-ROM ▶ CD Materials 13a–p, each sheet lists a course of action in partial steps. These steps have to be put in the right order (instructions: "Which order is the most suitable for…?"). For the first two actions "cooking pasta" (▶ CD Materials 13a), each of the eleven steps (A1–11) and for the action "birthday party" each of the five steps (B1–5) were written on a separate sheet of paper. At this point, only the latter two exercises (13a–b) are performed. The rest of the exercises of this series will be done in the restitution section of this module. The primary therapist explains the action (e.g., "We want to cook pasta"). Each participant – the co-therapist as well if the group is small – receives one or two sheets, each with one action step. The task is to put the separate action steps in the right sequence and to order the sheets accordingly. The goal is to reach a group consensus.

- **Concept Formation: Finding the Right Words**

As a preparation for the social-cognitive section of Module C, the compensation section on reasoning and problem solving concludes with coping strategies for improving concept formation in social contexts.

Examples of Key Questions

We usually think in words. Even if we have learned that understanding and expression using gestures and facial features are important factors in communication, we mostly exchange information with words in our everyday lives. Now we'll focus on speaking and writing:

- Do you immediately find the right words when you are in a conversation or when writing?
- Are there certain situations in which you are better at this? Or worse?
- Why is this? Do you have an explanation?

Participants' comments are collected on the flip chart. The aim is that the participants each describe concrete situations from their everyday lives illustrating personal strengths and weaknesses in finding words. If the group discussion finds that the difficulty in such concrete situations is primarily caused by mood, emotional state, or basic cognitive deficits, the therapists repeat the compensation strategies from the preceding section "Obstacles in goal realization". The focus here is on strategies for improving concept formation as a basis for a flexible use of language. For this purpose, ▶ CD Information Sheet 26 ("How can I better find the right words?") is available on the accompanying ▶ CD-ROM. Again, participants' first experiences are recorded by applying newly learned strategies in activating group exercises. The following exercises are available:

Collecting and Categorizing Concepts The co-therapist first writes a concept on the flip chart. Examples of this mostly include affectively stressful concepts such as therapeutic offers, medications, packing for moving house, and one's boss, but also affectively neutral concepts like packing for vacation, fruit, or recreational activities. Depending on the stress resistance of the group, it is usually best to start with an affectively neutral concept. Like the exercise "concept hierarchies" in the Integrated Psychological Therapy program (IPT, Roder et al. 2008a, 2011), the participants are now requested to name concepts that spontaneously occur to them upon seeing the written term (brainstorming). When at least 20 concepts have been compiled and written down, they are then assigned to categories and associated general terms in group discussion. Other comparable exercises that are also suitable are described in detail in the IPT manual (first subprogram; Roder et al. 2008a).

Activity In this exercise, the participants are assigned to two groups. If the number of participants is uneven, the co-therapist can also be included. The primary therapist writes a concept on a sheet of paper and gives it to the first group. The second group cannot see the written term. The first group now picks one or two members who try to describe the written concept verbally without using the word itself. This verbal description of the concept can also be accentuated with facial and physical gestures. The second group must now guess what the concept is. These group roles are then exchanged. The concept can also be described nonverbally or using drawings. It is again recommended that one start with affectively neutral concepts.

At this point, the card-sorting exercise "emotional concept formation" (materials 5a–h) from Module A can be repeated.

At the conclusion of the compensation section, the cognitive functions of reasoning and problem solving in social contexts are linked with perspective adoption (ToM). The following exercise is provided for this purpose:

On the basis of short detective stories, the group attempts to distinguish between "appearance" and "reality". By doing so, they attempt to arrive at the correct conclusion using existing facts and thus to the solution of the criminal case. Detective stories are available on the enclosed ▶ CD-ROM (▶ CD Worksheets 15a–d). In each of these stories, Inspector Frost and his team solve a case. The group reads one of the short stories together. At the end of the story, there are a few concrete questions about it. The objective is that each participant examines the facts and learns to argue about who the perpetrator could be.

2.3.3.1.3 Restitution

The restitution section contains both group and computer-based exercises. The goal is – as in previous modules – the repeated application of learned and individualized coping strategies in order to optimize functionality in the target area. Accordingly, participants receive ▶ CD Worksheet 4 ("My helpful strategies for…") and fill it out individually before each exercise.

The following will first describe the group exercises and then the computer-based exercises. When implementing these exercises, therapists should ensure that group and computer exercises are done alternately. This provides the participants with a stimulating treatment program in each session.

Group Exercises

The group exercises performed in the compensation section were meant merely to illustrate problems and coping strategies. These are now carried out completely using all available materials. The following group exercises described above are applied:

Group Exercises

- Problem solving
  - Matchstick exercise (▶ CD Materials 11)
  - Cube exercise (▶ CD Materials 12.1–20)
- Planning action
  - Which order is the most suitable? (▶ CD Materials 13c–p)
- Concept formation
  - Concept hierarchies (IPT, Roder et al. 2008a, 2011)
  - Collecting and categorizing concepts
  - "Activity"
  - Card-sorting exercise "emotional concept formation" (▶ CD Materials 5a-h)
  - Detective stories (▶ CD Worksheets 15a–d)

In order to involve visual stimuli in the process of concept formation as well as cognitive flexibility, the materials for the IPT card-sorting exercise (▶ CD Materials 1) and the "speed" card-sorting exercise (▶ CD Materials 2a–l) described in Modules A and B are used again, but with newly defined rules:

The group places at least ten randomly selected, well visible cards next to each other. The task is now to combine as many of these cards as possible using flexibly determinable criteria (homogenizing) – e.g., most of the cards of the IPT card-sorting exercise have a square, non-blue shape and a weekday. The cards which do not match must also be identified (discriminating) – e.g., cards with a round symbol without a weekday. The card-sorting exercise "speed" can be performed in the same way. The difficulty level can be increased gradually by increasing the number of cards. The object is that the participants make flexible use of the existing sort criteria of the cards and discuss them as a group.

Computer-Based Exercises

The didactic procedure follows that of the preceding module. The following well-tried CogPack exercises are available:

Problem Solving

SCALES This typical problem-solving exercise consists of three sub-exercises of increasing difficulty: a (weigh), b (balance easier), and c (balance harder). The participants start with sub-exercise a (weigh),which is the least challenging. All three sub-exercises are done.

LABYRINTHS This exercise contains nine sub-exercises (exercises a–i). In each, the time required to solve the task is measured. In the first four sub-exercises (exercises a–d), the labyrinths to be traversed increase gradually in complexity and difficulty. The objective is to animate the participants not only to work according to the principle of trial-and-error but also to develop strategies to solve them better and faster (e.g., first imagining the path backwards from finish to start, subdividing the labyrinth into sections). In the final sub-exercise (exercise i), the program automatically adjusts the difficulty level to previous results.

Reasoning

ANAGRAMS In this exercise, a correct word must be formed from a nonsense word by rearranging the letters (e.g., OSER to ROSE). Again, the point is to develop strategies for solving the task (e.g., forming syllables, using vowels).

GUESSWORDS As in the exercise "anagrams", a target word must be found given a paraphrase (e.g., target word "clock": "shows us the time"). As opposed to the "anagram" exercise, the letters of the target word are not provided, only the number of letters by means of placeholders. Once again, the participants are encouraged not simply to try out the entire alphabet but to develop strategies (vowels, frequently used consonants like R and S, or forming syllables).

CONCEPTS In this typical exercise on verbal concept formation, the objective is to find one concept among six that does not match the others. There are two variants, each with twelve tasks.

CONFUSION (Sub-exercises "Puzzles") In this exercise, only the puzzle sub-exercises (j–p) are recommended. Again, the participants should first develop strategies (which squares go together, which squares should be expected at the upper edge of the picture (e.g., sky) and which at the bottom edge).

Group and computer-based exercises are repeated in alternation. After each exercise block, difficulties and successful experiences are discussed and analyzed. On the basis of ▶ CD Information Sheets 21–26 and the individualized compensation strategies derived from it on ▶ CD Worksheet 4 ("My helpful strategies for …"), the group discusses personal benefits and difficulties they experienced.

At the end of the restitution section, the participants review and correct the self-assessments made at the start of

Module C regarding their performance in the target areas on ▶ CD Worksheets 12 ("How well can I reason in my everyday life?") and 13 ("How how can I solve problems?").

2.3.3.1.4 In Vivo Exercises and Independent Exercises

Compensation strategies for optimizing reasoning and problem solving performance have now been learned in interventions and practiced in group or computer exercises. These strategies are now applied individually by means of in vivo exercises or independent exercises. As a rule, it requires several sessions or weeks to realize the individual goals for coping with everyday problems that were found in the compensation section. The problems are now more complex (e.g., in the vocational and recreational domains). It should also be taken into consideration that the following module (D) is highly demanding for the participants. Overstraining the participants with too many tasks should be avoided at all costs. If there are highly motivated participants, therapists can discuss other everyday problems with them individually and develop corresponding solution strategies, which they can then try to implement between sessions.

2.3.3.2 Social-Cognitive Intervention Area: Social Schema

Module C: Social-Cognitive Intervention Area: Social Schemas

1. Introduction
   - Definition: automatic patterns of thought and behavior (social schema), social roles and rules, prejudices
   - Self-perception in the target area
   - Resource-oriented individual profile in the target area
   - Connection to self and everyday life: case vignette
2. Compensation
   - Identifying social roles and rules
   - Recognizing one's own nonconforming behavior patterns
   - Dealing with stigmatization
   - Social action sequences (scripts)
3. Restitution
   - Habituation of learned coping strategies in repeated group exercises on social scripts and video sequences
4. In vivo exercises and independent exercises
   - Transfer of individualized coping strategies to concrete, everyday situations

Tips

- Infrastructure: group therapy room, flip chart, projector
- Therapy materials: ▶ CD Information Sheets 27–29, ▶ CD Worksheets 5,16–17, ▶ CD Vignette 13, ▶ CD e-Materials 7–8; commercial videos (commercially available)
- Didactics: structured group discussion

2.3.3.2.1 Introductory Sessions

▪ Definition of the Target Area

The interventions about social schemas refer directly to the functions of reasoning, problem solving, and planning from the neurocognitive section of Module C. Here, the therapy targets are action sequences and problems in social contexts (social scripts). While goal-oriented, consciously controlled thought and behavior was discussed in the implementation of problem-solving and planning steps in the neurocognitive section, now the focus is on mostly automatic social patterns that directly control behavior. Individual attitudes and habits make it possible (automatically) to process information perceived in social situations quickly and effortlessly and to behave appropriately. Social knowledge concerning the norms and roles regulating society and behavior is applied automatically in everyday social actions.

But this automatic, unconscious use of social knowledge is interrupted if something unexpected or surprising occurs in a situation or when a social situation is considered to be especially important. This can be seen again and again in social situations that are felt to be straining by patients with schizophrenia, resulting in nonconforming behavior. Patients' personal experiences also often involve the topics of exclusion, lack of understanding, stigmatization, and "being different". This highly relevant subject matter will be dealt with in the second part of the module.

The initial objective is to explain and define the concept – an abstract one for most participants – of social schemas. The concept of schemas will be replaced in the following by the more everyday terms of "automatic thought" or "behavior patterns". When introducing this subject, therapists should maintain a link to previous therapy content in the way of a recurrent theme within the program.

Introduction Example

At the beginning, we were concerned with reasoning, problem solving, and planning actions. When dealing with planning solutions to problems, we learned to consider separate action steps consciously, to analyze and implement them, and finally to check whether we are satisfied with the outcome. Now we are dealing with how we behave in everyday life when we don't think about it much. In any given situation, our behavior

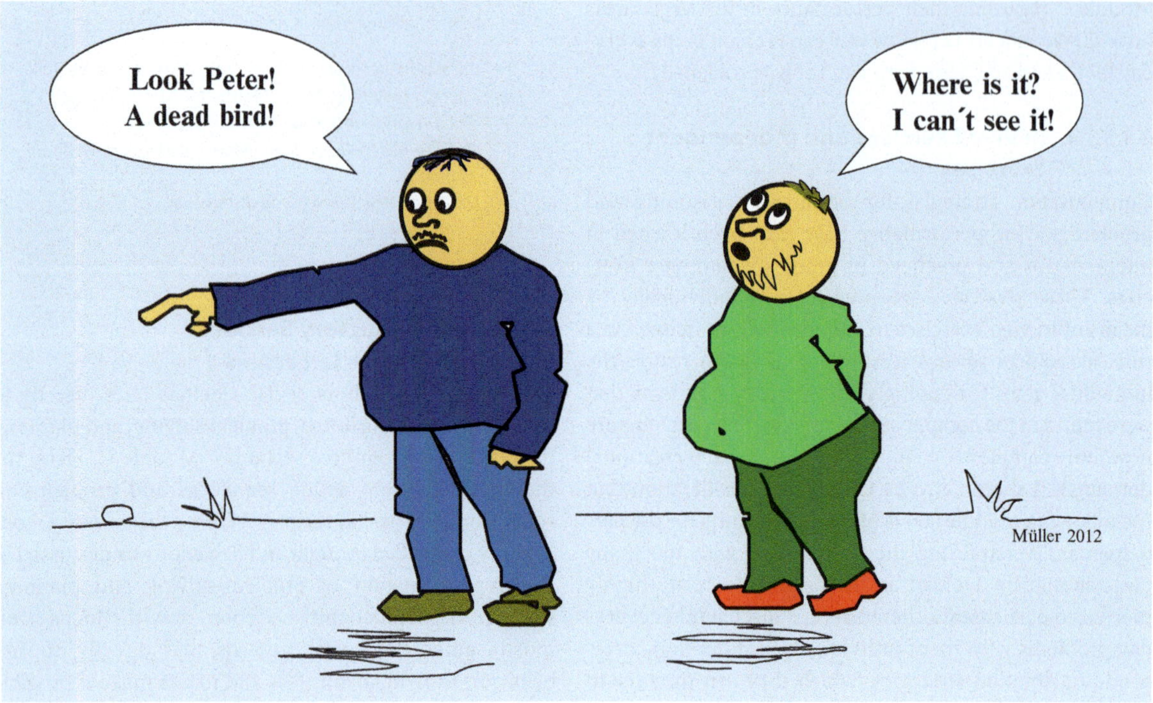
Look Peter!
A dead bird!
Where is it?
I can´t see it!
Müller 2012

Fig. 2.22 Social schemas: automatic processes

is usually spontaneous, quick, and effortless. We don't need to think about it, and it requires no effort. Our experiences with comparable situations and the thought and behavior patterns we acquire from them are helpful here. You could say that we're all "creatures of habit"; we automatically think and behave in the same way again and again. We all have contact with other people, here in this group for example. For this to work, our thought and behavior patterns are oriented towards social rules, norms, and roles. These determine what we are allowed to do and what we had best not do. Or in other words: Internalized social roles and rules determine how we behave with one another.

See Fig. 2.22 for an example of automatic processes and the activation of social schemas.

The following behavioral experiments serve to illustrate social rules:

Greeting The primary therapist announces a short behavioral exercise. She or the co-therapist then approaches a participant, greets him amicably and offers her hand. As a rule, the participant addressed reciprocates the greeting and shakes the therapist's hand. The group then explores why the participant shook the therapist's hand – whether the participant thought about it or whether this reaction took place automatically.

The aim of these exercises is for the group to identify the underlying social roles and rules that led to the automatic action. Participants' comments are recorded on the flip chart. Automatic thought patterns (schemas) are often worded as behavioral prompts in this context. For example: "You have to be friendly!", "You have to show interest in others!", "You have to respond to a greeting – that's simply how it's done!", but also "If a group leader addresses someone in the group, that person has to participate!"

Additionally, the following exercise can also be used to demonstrate prototypical thought patterns. This experiment, often utilized in social psychology, is presented here in a modified, milder form to avoid the possibility of strain.

The primary therapist tells the following story:

A father and son are involved in a car crash. Both have been injured, but they are not in critical condition. Both have broken legs and are being driven by ambulance to the nearest hospital to be operated on. In the emergency department of the hospital, the father is rolled into one of the operating rooms and the son into the other, where they are already expected. In the son's operating room, a member of the surgical team approaches him and cries out: 'Oh my god, that's my son!'

The primary therapist now asks the group who said the last statement.

Very few participants arrive at the answer that it could be the mother of the injured party. Behind this lies the assumption that a surgeon is usually male.

For further illustration and definition of social norms, ▶ CD Information Sheet 27 ("Social rules and roles") is available on the accompanying ▶ CD-ROM.

▪ Promoting Self-Perception in the Cognitive Target Area

On the basis of ▶ CD Information Sheet 27, the participants are asked with what social rules and roles they are confronted in their everyday lives. Their statements are recorded on the flip chart. The therapists should take heed that prohibitions, laws, and rules stipulated by law or religious writings are not the only one's mentioned. In addition, the group should focus on everyday, usually automated action sequences in social contexts, called "social scripts". Typical, oft-mentioned examples from the everyday lives of participants include:

- **The social role as a restaurant guest:** recognizing a restaurant with associated features (table, chairs, menus and beverage lists), entering, seeking a table and asking for a menu, choosing a meal and drink, ordering from the waiter, consuming, asking for the bill, paying, leaving, etc.
- **The role as a customer shopping at the supermarket:** making a shopping list, looking for and finding a supermarket, seeking required products on the shopping list and perhaps asking for information with an employee, recognizing desired products on the shelves and placing them in the shopping cart, putting all the products on the checkout belt, paying and bagging the purchased products, etc.
- **Role as a girlfriend meeting her best friend:** greetings usually follow the same ritual: a reciprocal kiss with the question "How are you?", "So so." "And how about you?" "Good. Where are we going?" etc.

Other common examples also concern roles and rules in interpersonal relationships or in participants' encounters in the vocational, residential, and recreational domains.

As in previous intervention areas, the goal here is also to promote a more discerning self-perception so that the latter can be optimized in the course of the intervention. First the participants are asked in which of the examples mentioned their own (automated) thought and behavior patterns function better, i.e., in which situations the rules of a specific social role can be complied with well and in which not. And finally, what internal and external influences might the thought and behavior patterns in the above situations/roles are based on? The discussion also takes into account the effects of alertness, mood, and emotional and situational strain as discussed in previous modules.

The participants can use the following behavioral experiment in order to perceive consciously automatic actions:

Consciously Controlled Walking The primary therapist asks one or two of the participants whether they are willing to walk in front of the other participants from one side of the group room to the other. The participants are asked whether this motion sequence was difficult to perform, which they presumably answer in the negative. In the second step, the participants are now told to walk once again, but this time in a consciously controlled manner. Specifically, the participants are asked to comment on the walking process out loud in such a way that for each step they say in advance which muscle contraction and motion they now intend to perform. For example: "I will now contract my thigh muscle to raise my right leg. I must then bend forward slightly in order to place my right foot on the floor in the planned direction of movement about 50 cm in front of my left foot. I will also use my back muscles in the process for maintaining equilibrium, and I have to tighten my calf muscle a bit in order to support myself after setting down my right foot..." Generally, every participant has to make the utmost effort to walk in such a way. In other words, conscious control of automated actions is quite difficult because it is unfamiliar and new.

In conclusion, the participants are instructed first to assess their own ability concerning how well they are able to utilize their own thought and action patterns for practicing social roles in everyday life. For this purpose, each participant fills out ▶ CD Worksheet 16 ("How well can I deal with social rules?"), which is discussed analogously to the method described above.

▪ Case Vignette

One case vignette is available on the subject of social schemas on the accompanying ▶ CD-ROM (▶ CD Vignette 13: "By bike to Café Adonis"). The vignettes are read section-by-section as described above. The participants are then asked whether they have had similar experiences in their everyday lives. The contributions of the participants are again recorded on the flip chart.

▪ Prejudices

Thought and behavior patterns stemming from social rules and roles can also lead to excessively rigid attitudes. In the following, the group will focus on this using the term "prejudices" It is important to show the participants that no one – including the participants and therapists alike – is immune to prejudices. The following optional topic of stigmatization is often associated with stress. Accordingly, prejudices should be introduced in a playful and humorous way to reduce the associated stress potential.

Introduction Example

Attitudes are based on our thought and behavior patterns and help us directly in orienting ourselves in everyday life. We use attitudes to define and categorize others and ourselves. Especially when we are unfamiliar with something and start to become fearful of that unknown thing, sometimes we tend to distance ourselves from it. If we do this again and again in the same way and are also influenced by others in the process, prejudices can arise. Prejudices always entail value judgments. These can be communicated in the guise of humor, in jokes for example. Everybody is familiar with jokes about women or about men, about people from different countries, about the outer appearances of people (such as blonde jokes), or about certain professions.

Assuming that patients with schizophrenia need unambiguous, clear, easily comprehensible statements to orient themselves by, many specialists avoid the use of jokes with this clientele. This approach often ignores that humor is especially relaxing and thus can reduce stress and anxiety. Furthermore, jokes made by the participants, sometimes overstepping "good manners", can be exploited within the group dynamics as examples of violating social rules. The following is presented as a possible example. A 60-year-old woman participating in an INT group told this joke during an in vivo exercise:

An older married couple, both 60 years of age, was walking together one Sunday in the forest. Both of them looked happy, were satisfied and enjoyed being together. Suddenly a fairy appeared. She watched the married couple, and took visible pleasure in their happiness. The fairy said: 'Hello. I'm very happy that you both make such a happy couple. Therefore I would like to bestow a gift. Each of you can make one wish. What will you wish for?' The wife answered spontaneously: 'That is very generous of you. I wish for two tickets for a world tour. One for me and one for my husband.' The fairy waved her magic wand and instantly the wife was holding two tickets in her hand. Then the fairy turned to the husband and told him to make haste, as she still had much to do. The husband was having a hard time deciding. After a long delay, he finally said: 'Fine, know I know what I want. I wish for a wife who is 20 years younger than me!' The fairy answered: 'If that is your greatest wish, so be it.' Again the fairy waved her magic wand, and the husband instantly turned into an 80-year-old man!

This or similar examples can be used together with the participants to help identify and question both widespread prejudices and one's own personal prejudices. Possible key questions for group discussion using a concrete include the following:

Examples of Key Questions

- Why do we like to tell discriminating jokes, blonde jokes for example?
- How do blonde jokes come about?
- Why do we laugh at them?
- How does a blonde woman feel when she hears this? Does she feel excluded?
- Are blonde people really dumb and naive?
- Why do many women dye their hair blond?
- Are prejudices based on facts or ungrounded assumptions?

Using concrete examples volunteered by participants, the group discusses underlying thought patterns and expectations (e.g., a blonde has to be attractive and sexy, but somewhat naive) as well as associated social roles and rules (e.g., a blonde embodies a role of women which is archaic but nonetheless still occupies our minds as thought patterns: the attractive and desirable, yet uneducated woman, who knows how to use her charms). The primary therapist leads the discussion so that participants can introduce examples not only of their own use of prejudices but also of experiences as targets/victims of prejudice.

Participants with longer illness durations in particular may also mention experiences of exclusion resulting from the still widespread stigmatization of mental illness, especially schizophrenia and psychosis. Experiences of exclusion can lead to massive damage to self-worth and to social withdrawal. Accordingly, therapists listen to such experiences in an affirming way. Possible ways to deal adaptively with such experiences and especially associated prevention strategies will be discussed in the next compensation section. If the topic of stigmatization is broached, it is of central importance for the time being to make the persons concerned aware that, in many situations in social life, the illness plays only a secondary role. In such cases, the patients can do something themselves to prevent negative consequences stemming from their environment with appropriate modes of thought and behavior.

2.3.3.2.2 Compensation

Based on the topics introduced in the introductory section, coping strategies are now developed which can be applied first in group exercises. In the course of the interventions on social schemas, the therapeutic approach generally applied during the INT procedure manifests itself even more clearly than in preceding INT modules: Largely automatic, action-directing processes from the participants' everyday lives are identified, reflected on, and modified before they are habituated in the group via incremental practice and re-automated in everyday life (▪ Fig. 2.23). From the therapist's perspective, this means that action-directing processes in social contexts that are mostly automated and unconsciously controlled are reflected on and modified during the treatment. Yet this requires a linguistic interpretation of habitual behaviors in order to reflect on them and modify them if need be. The success of many behavioral modifications ultimately

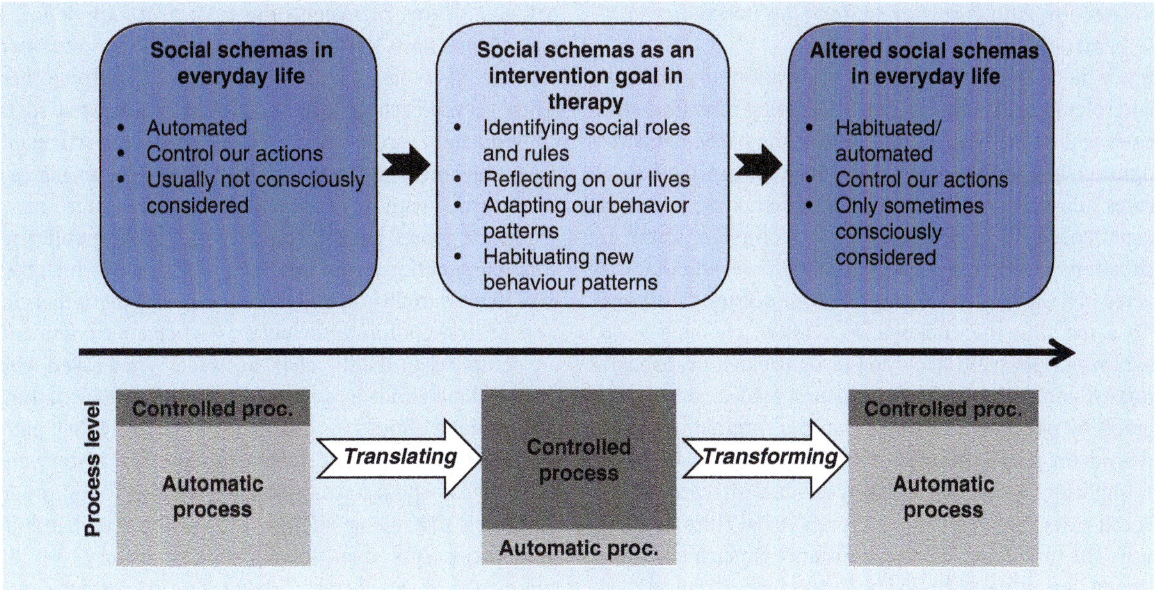

Fig. 2.23 Intervention goal: social schemas (social roles and rules), Therapy process

depends on how well they can be habituated and transferred to the daily life of the patients.

Identifying Social Roles and Rules

The concrete situations already volunteered in the introductory section by the participants – situations in which individual thought and behavior patterns have become rigid – are now expanded upon in the group. However, the focus now lies more heavily on the underlying social roles and rules.

Examples of Key Questions

- In which situations and in what personal experiences did I have the feeling that a person should behave exactly in one way and not another, that a person should say exactly this and nothing else?
- How did this make me feel?
- Was it easy for me to follow this? Or did I have the feeling that other people don't understand me (because I'm different)?

The first objective is to collect concrete situations from the lives of the participants. For example:

- If someone greets me amiably, then I should also return the greeting.
- If my boss orders me to do something, I should listen carefully and show him that I have understood what he expects of me or ask questions if I did not understand.
- If the pedestrian lights are on red, I have to wait like the other pedestrians until it changes to green.
- If someone smiles at me, I should smile back.

The last example clarifies the distinction with the social cognition "attribution style", which is first addressed in Module D. Here the focus is on recognizing social rules and roles, not on explaining why the other person does or says something. Contributions associated with attribution are registered, but therapists should refer to Module D for further exploration of the topic.

For better illustration and i to give participants the chance to experience the effect of social rules and roles, previously mentioned situations can be acted out in a role play.

One participant mentioned the following example: "When someone asks me something, I can't answer!" The primary therapist now asks a participant in a previously announced role play to solve a very difficult task ("What is the square root of 169?" or "What is the capital of Nigeria?"). The roles should initially be clarified: in this interaction, there is the role of the questioner (primary therapist) and the role of the person addressed. Also, social rules which are decisive for the person addressed are identified: "When I am asked something, I should give an answer, even if I say or gesture that I don't know the answer." In this example it is also recommended to discuss and reduce the level of expectation: "Nobody can expect the other person to know or understand everything!" or "I don't have to know the answer to everything!"

The goal is that the participants understand that misinterpreted social rules and consequently inappropriate behavior can lead to unnecessary emotional strain.

Recognizing Own Nonconforming Behavior Patterns

From the patient's perspective, the violation of social rules and roles is a central issue. In the following therefore, strategies will be developed that can help the participants recognize when their own behavior threatens to violate social rules in a concrete situation. Again, first social situations experienced by group members are compiled. These are situations in which a participant had the feeling that they acted in a way that was wrong or not understood by others. To assist this, the enclosed ▶ CD-ROM contains ▶ CD Information Sheet 28 ("How do I recognize that my behavior doesn't conform to rules?"), which is read together paragraph by paragraph. Further strategies originating during discussion should be noted on ▶ CD Information Sheet 28. It is important also to discuss the individual interpretation of social rules. Not everyone interprets social rules the same way. The time-tested closeness-distance experiment makes a good illustration of (individually interpreted) social rules:

Nearness-Distance Experiment

One of the group leaders approaches one of the participants. The participant was previously instructed to say "stop" when the distance to the group leader becomes uncomfortably close. This closeness-distance experiment is now repeated in different ways. Particular stress is placed on the influence of gender (woman-woman, man-woman), one's role in the group (therapist-participant, participant-participant), the level of mutual acquaintance (I'm familiar with this person and I'm known her for a long time, or not), and age (the same age or different ages) as well as combinations of these factors. "Do the factors described affect my feeling of distance?", "How do I recognize, which I come too close to someone?", "How do I recognize, when someone comes too close to me?", and "How can I distance myself if someone comes too close?"

This nearness-distance experiment makes it clear that the intervention on social rules is not exclusively concerned with promoting behavior that conforms to rules as much as possible. The intervention also deals with but being able to distance oneself in a socially acceptable way when others violate rules. The task of the therapist here is to prevent the participants from demanding too much of themselves, thereby circumventing excessive strain. The objective is to give the participants more self-confidence to behave and think in a way that is socially appropriate and conforms to rules.

Dealing with Stigmatization

Connecting these topics with participants' everyday lives has a higher emotional potential than usual, which should be taken into account. Whether and in what form this topic can be broached depends to a great extent on the patients' degree of insight and treatment experience. If participants have less insight, the goal of the group interventions is to sensitize them to how they affect others when they breach certain social norms and what social consequences can result from this. Yet many participants are highly interested in the topic of stigmatization, since it is concerned with real experiences from daily life.

In the group, participants are first asked to volunteer concrete situations from their everyday lives in which they experienced exclusion and rejection as a result of their illness or non-conformal behavior. Participants' comments are compiled on the flip chart as usual. When asked what can be done about it, a common answer is that nothing can be done about it – especially when the other party knows something about the patient's medical history and associated hospital stays. Thus the main focus of this intervention is distancing oneself from others, i.e., handling information on one's own medical history. ▶ CD Information Sheets 29a–b ("Being able to distance ourselves: easier said than done") are available for this purpose on the accompanying ▶ CD-ROM. Taking the concrete example of a previous hospital stay, various strategies for handling associated information are discussed and illustrated, partly via role play. The focus is both on one's own willingness and confidence to apply a strategy in a concrete situation and considering which strategy is promising and with whom.

Examples of Key Questions

- Am I obligated to provide information about where I was in the last few weeks?
- To whom do I feel more obligated? To whom less?
- What do I trust myself to do (in which situation)?
- What are the pros and cons of the different strategies?
- What consequences does each of these strategies have for me and for others?
- What do I think and feel in the process? Does it influence my behavior?
- One of the group leaders plays a curious neighbor who wants to know where a person, played by a participant, has been in the last 2 weeks (hospital stay). The said participant must now take over the conversation and change the topic. For example, he or she could talk about work, a sports match, the weather, etc. The goal is to distract from the initial topic "Where were you in the last couple of weeks?" and to replace it with another topic.

In the final step of this intervention, possible coping methods of distancing oneself are individualized. For this purpose, each participant fills out ▶ CD Worksheet 17 ("Which distancing strategy is good for me?"): First,

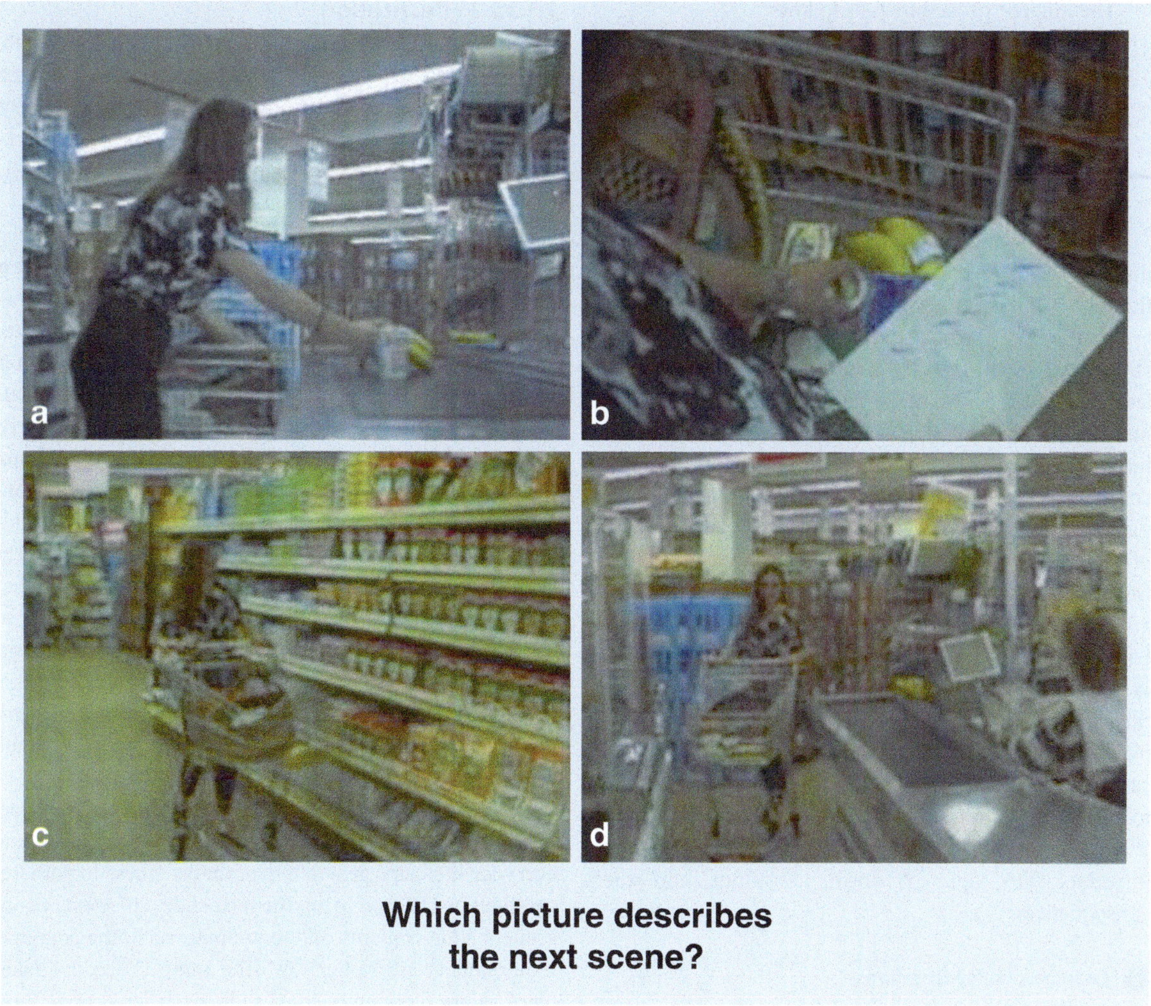

Fig. 2.24 Example of a visually represented social action sequence (script) (Photos: J. Funke, Psychological Institute Heidelberg, with kind permission)

participants write down possible individual advantages and disadvantages for each coping strategy. They also note with whom these strategies are applicable. This individual information is compiled in the subsequent group discussion. Each participant adds the information of other participants on his worksheet insofar as it is personally relevant. This worksheet now can serve as an orientation aid for every participant, summarizing the individualized coping repertoire.

Action Sequences (Scripts)

At the conclusion of the compensation section, the group focuses on action sequences and problems in social contexts. This intervention bridges back to the automated thought and behavior patterns addressed already in the introductory section. It covers the residential, vocational, and recreational domains as well as interpersonal relationships in the everyday lives of the participants. The intervention also serves as a preparation for the exercises in the following restitution section.

As an introduction, participant experiences of social action sequences already compiled in previous interventions should be updated, summarized, and supplemented if necessary. The key question here is: "How does the social rule (norm) require that I behave in this everyday social situation?" For illustration, simple action sequences, called "social scripts" (Schank and Abelson 1977) are used as initial examples. These generally exert a low level of strain on the participants. A total of twelve picture series on social scripts are available on the enclosed ► CD-ROM (► CD e-Materials 7 and 8). The 12 picture series contain a total of 78 slides each with four photos (a total of 312 photos). At this point it is sufficient to utilize 2–3 slides as examples. The entire picture series will be used in the following restitution section. Figure 2.24 contains an example of a sequence of scenes in a supermarket.

The didactic procedure is as follows:

The four pictures contained in ◘ Fig. 2.24 are presented to the group on a slide. The group's task is self-explanatory: The four pictures need to be put in the proper order. This order has to be justified in the ensuing group discussion using objective facts (target stimuli).

There are always participants who find it easy to discover a correct sequence. This signifies that their thought/behavior-guiding social schemas are appropriate to the situation. The objective is to make them aware of the strategies they use. On the other hand, participants with less pronounced resources in this area often require instructions and orientation aids. For this, therapists can have recourse to ▶ CD Information Sheet 25 ("From a complicated action to small action steps") to review action planning. But the point here is to make participants aware of automated action sequences (schemas), which differs from controlled planning of separate action steps. The group is now focused on the analysis of individual images. Later they will determine the objective of the action – in ◘ Fig. 2.24, it is shopping and paying for required items in the supermarket – and the action's starting point (attending to a shopping list). For further assistance, the situation can be performed in a role play as well. This can help both to establish a connection to the participants' personal experience of themselves and their everyday lives and to introduce the topic of norm deviations and their consequences.

Examples of Key Questions

- What is the usual course of action (when shopping)? Is there a series of actions one should adhere to? Do I always do that?
- What could happen if someone didn't act according to the norm? Would it attract attention?
- What happens when I don't act according to the norm? For example, when I put my purchases directly into my pockets in the supermarket and only take them out again at the checkout instead of using one of the shopping baskets or carts provided?
- Does this have consequences for me? Which?

The aim is to encourage participant self-reflection about the influence of social rules on one's own, often automated behavior. This should finally lead to the insight that behavior that conforms to rules helps to reduce stress-inducing experiences. Strategies for better recognizing one's own nonconforming behavior and for distancing oneself against rule violations made by others have already been discussed. These will now be rehearsed in the following restitution section.

2.3.3.2.3 Restitution

The restitution section is organized in three stages: In the first two stages, previously introduced action sequences (scripts) are analyzed by means of visually depicted everyday situations. In the third stage, video materials will be employed to identify social schemas.

Stage 1

The intervention of the first stage has the lowest level of difficulty and emotional activation. Six picture series depicting everyday actions are available on the enclosed ▶ CD-ROM as didactic tools. The topics are: "Getting up in the morning", "Telephone booth", "Supermarket", "Restaurant", "Coffee machine", and "Bus ride". Each series of pictures consists of ten slides each with four photos (▶ CD e-Materials 7a1–f10). In this group exercise, only one slide at a time is projected on the screen. The first slide always shows a starting situation in four images. The participants' task is first to describe objective facts that they see in the pictures. Following this, assumptions can be made regarding what kind of action might be occurring. On each slide is also the question "Which picture describes the next scene?" This means that the group has to agree upon which order the four pictures of the first slide should be put. The last picture of the series then gives an indication of how the depicted action might further develop. Connecting to patients' experiences of themselves and everyday life helps generate hypotheses. These hypotheses can then be checked using the next slide. Since every subsequent slide contains only one photo each, the cognitive requirements are rather low. The same procedure takes place before showing the next slide. Each series of pictures consists of ten slides each with one new picture (action step) proceeding from the previous slide. Thus, each picture series consists of 13 visually depicted action steps. Concluding the exercise, the participants are asked to find an overarching title for the visually represented action. In order to lower the level of difficulty, the number of slides can also be reduced if necessary. Since the image content and topics are identical to those of the second stage, it is recommended that only half of the series is used, leaving the rest of the series to be employed later after introducing the second stage.

Stage 2

Now and then, there are patients with good resources who need little effort to master the stage 1 exercises. As stated in the compensation section however, the objective is to make them conscious of the strategies they use and to discuss them in the group. This is also done from the point of view that the better one can remember the previous scenes of the picture series, the less effort (capacity) is needed to assess the next scene adequately. Knowledge about the past gives confidence in judging the present (feeling of consistency). This is plainly visible when the previous scene suddenly cannot be recalled after changing slides or the difficulty of the task is increased. In this case, the more intensive process of describing and interpreting should be activated in order to find the correct solution. One becomes less sure of oneself and requires more capacity. In order to illustrate this to the participants, the group works through the six picture series of ▶ CD e-Materials 8a1–f3 in the second stage. Each of these picture series contains three slides, each again with four photos. As with ▶ CD e-Materials 7 of stage 1, the first picture of each series portrays a starting situation. The point again is to put the pictures in a correct order so as to identify the fourth and last picture. As opposed to the materials used in stage 1, now the next slide does not repeat any of the previously shown pictures. This means that each new slide contains four new pictures. There is therefore no reference to the visual cue stimuli of the previous scene. Due to the lack of a visual memory aid, the capacity requirement is also increased. Participants have to engage in processes of description and interpretation to a greater degree. The group members are thus required to give a correct ordering of the four pictures for each slide. Every suggestion is noted on the flip chart. As a rule, several alternative suggestions of action sequences are compiled. Participants must now defend their suggestions against other alternatives using objective facts and logical conclusions. Again, the point is to replace assertions with the interpretation of facts (e.g., "This picture was taken before entering the supermarket, because the shopping cart is still empty.") In order to check the result and to support memory of information contained on previous slides, the therapist team switches back to previous slides if required. If one of the six picture series has been completed and the entire action sequence (divided over 3 slides/12 pictures) successfully guessed, then the group summarizes the entire action with a concise title. For support and illustration, individual segments of the action can be presented again in the form of a role play. As described in the compensation section, the activity concludes by encouraging the participants to connect the content with their personal, everyday lives.

? Examples of Key Questions

- Have you experienced such situations?
- How do you behave?
- Do you know immediately what is required of you?
- What happens when you don't meet that requirement?
- Does this have consequences?
- How do you feel and how do you react?

▪ Stage 3

On a more complex level, the group leader utilizes film excerpts to illustrate social schemas. As in past modules, commercially available films are used. The goal is to watch succinct (and often exaggeratedly played) scenes together with the group, in which everyday action sequences, pronounced thought and behavior patterns, prejudices, or rule violations and norm deviations are depicted. It is up to the therapist team to monitor the level of strain and complexity of the selected film material and to estimate its compatibility with the group. It is recommended that one start with less demanding and clearly interpretable content, then raising the difficulty gradually. As described in detail in Module B, this intervention is also based exclusively on short film excerpts, not on complete films. As opposed to Module B, analyses of the film sequences are not primarily focused on adopting the perspectives of the characters (ToM) but on identifying action-directing social schemas in addition to social rules. The characters may follow these rules more or less or – in comedies, for example – break them frequently. In order to differentiate from the social-cognitive interventions in Module D, justifying actions (attribution) is also not stressed here.

As a rule, the same films can be employed here as were listed in Module B. It is also possible to work on the same film scene repeatedly, but from different perspectives, e.g., as an intervention on perspective adoption in Module B, for recognizing social rules and roles in Module C, and finally with a focus on attribution in Module D. The list has been supplemented with other films:

- "Analyze This", with Robert De Niro and Billy Crystal, USA 1999
- "Analyze That", with Robert De Niro and Billy Crystal, USA 2002
- "There's Something About Mary", with Cameron Diaz and Ben Stiller, USA 1998
- "What about Bob?", with Bill Murray and Richard Dreifuss, USA 1991
- "Groundhog Day", with Bill Murray and Andie MacDowell, USA 1993
- "A Beautiful Mind", with Russell Crowe, USA 2001
- "Elling", with Per Christian Ellefsen and Sven Nordin, Norway/Sweden 2001
- "Mors Elling", with Per Christian Ellefsen and Grethe Nordra, Norwegen/Schweden 2003
- "As Good as it Gets", with Jack Nicholson and Helen Hunt, USA 1997

With the exception of "Groundhog Day", each film addresses with topic of psychiatry and psychotherapy in a broader sense. However, only scenes in which situation comedy is in the foreground are recommended. Examples of nonconforming behavior can be found in scenes like

"Butcher's platter at the restaurant" or "Neighbor's help" from the film "Elling" or Chapter 8 from the film "Analyze this", in which two Mafiosi appear unannounced at a medical practice.

The objective of this group exercise is to sensitize participants with regard to the importance of social norms as well as the consequences of deviations from norms. The costs and uses of social norms (excessive conformity vs. being crazy) can also be discussed. Therapists can vary the degree of self-perception and emotional activation by controlling and structuring the self-reference made by the participants.

? Less Emotionally Activating Key Questions

- How does the actor feel in the scene?
- How do the other people react?
- How might the actor feel as a result of the reaction of the other people?

Work on social cognition remains on a more distanced, less emotionally activating level here. However, the therapist can increase the level of emotional activation with corresponding key questions.

? Key Questions for Increasing the Level of Activation

- Have I had such experiences in my everyday life?
- What would I do?
- Have I also reacted like the actor in the scene?
- Can I identify with the actors in the film?
- With which person do I identify the most?

At this point, it is important to stress the aspect of coping.

? Key Questions on the Aspect of Coping

- How do I cope when I receive negative reactions?
- Do I even perceive them?
- What could I change?

The scene "Flirt" from the film "Beautiful Mind" is also suitable. In this scene, the main actor communicates his sexual intentions to a woman very directly and is slapped as a result. Participants' personal identification is probably the most emotionally activating in this scene.

At the conclusion of this intervention section, the participants supplement or correct the self-assessments they made of their skills in dealing with social schemas on ► CD Worksheet 16 ("How well can I deal with social rules?").

2.3.3.2.4 In Vivo Exercises and Independent Exercises

Group in vivo exercises can help participants reflect on the effect of social schemas on everyday human behavior, recognize social norms along with associated laws and prohibitions, and analyze individual habits (thought and behavior patterns). Any kind of group activity is suitable for this, for example a visit to a cafeteria, a walk through town, or a target oriented activity. The objective is to help enable the participants to experience the influence of social schemas outside of the therapy room. Social roles and rules and their consequences can be discussed on the basis of social events that occur during the in vivo exercise: How do we behave and that do we think, e.g., when a pedestrian light suddenly changes to red, when we place an order at the cafeteria for the whole group, when we buy something at the kiosk, when we are addressed during a walk by someone in the group with whom we hardly have any personal contact, when we are in a restaurant for the first time and urgently need to use the toilet, etc. In addition to this rather analytically self-reflexive activity, participants should also do an in vivo exercise to try out coping strategies in everyday situations, e.g., strategies for recognizing one's own nonconforming behavior.

In addition, participants are given individual independent exercises (homework) at this point. For many participants, it is initially easier to identify their own thought and behavior patterns (e.g., "I noticed that I always go the same way to work") and social rules (e.g., "I have to buy a ticket before I ride the bus!"). Another objective is to motivate the participants to apply the compensation strategies they have learned, e.g., strategies for distancing themselves from others. As usual, ► CD Worksheet 5 ("Independent exercise") is filled out in preparation for each independent exercise (and each in vivo exercise). The subsequent discussion follows the formula described in the previous intervention unit.

2.3.4 INT Module D

The neurocognitive section of Module D focuses on working memory. As opposed to the functions of verbal and visual memory discussed in Module B, working memory is defined as an executive function. It is necessary for processes of decision making, defining goals, problem solving, and conscious selective perception. In contrast to the concept of vigilance from Module A, which described sustained attention in cases of understimulation, the stress-inducing effect of sensory overload is in the foreground of interventions on working memory. As a result, the level of emotional strain is higher than in previous neurocognitive interventions in the INT program. As opposed to short-term memory (Module B), the purpose of working memory is to "work with information". This information is made available in memory for goal-oriented processing whenever required.

INT also focuses on processes of selective attention in social contexts in the social-cognitive area of attribution styles. The treatment is centered on the perception of individual stress-generating situations and on developing adaptive coping strategies. Distorted causal attributions (attributional bias) are often the basis for persisting delusional symptoms, which are experienced by the sufferer as stress-inducing and emotionally straining in daily life. For this reason, the social-cognitive section of this module concludes with interventions that actively promote stress management and emotion regulation.

2.3.4.1 Neurocognitive Intervention Area: Working Memory

Module D: Neurocognitive Intervention Area: Working Memory

1. Introduction: working memory
   - Definition of working memory: control center for working with memory, distractibility and selective attention
   - Self-perception in the target area (cognitive profile)
   - Reference to everyday life and self: case vignette
   - Influential factor: overstimulation
2. Compensation
   - Learning and individualizing coping strategies:
     - Dealing with distraction and overstimulation in cases of sensory overload
     - Action rituals and behavior modification
     - Adaptability between several actions
     - Preventing distraction during a conversation
3. Restitution
   - Habituation of learned coping strategies:
     - Repetition of group exercises
     - Computer exercises
4. In vivo exercises and independent exercises
   - Transfer of individualized coping strategies to concrete, everyday situations

Tips

- Infrastructure: group therapy and computer rooms, flip chart, digital projector
- Therapy materials: ► CD Information Sheets 2, 30–34, ► CD Worksheets 4–5, 18–20, ► CD Vignettes 14–15, ► CD Materials 2, 14–18, ► CD e-Materials 9
- CogPack programs: SEARCH, CONNECT, MONEY, COLORS&LABELS, INTERFERENCE, LINESEGMENTS, PIESEGMENTS, NUMBERS, GEOMETRY, SEQUENCE, NEWorNOT, ONtheROAD, READING, GEOGRAPHY
- Didactics: structured group discussion, group exercises, computer exercises

2.3.4.1.1 Introductory Sessions

▪ Definition of the Target Area: Working Memory

Most participants are unaware of the concept of working memory. A definition would thus appear to be essential. It is recommended to paraphrase the concept of working memory as "working with memory". This definition should preserve the distinction from short-term and long-term memory as well as from vigilance during understimulation. In addition, therapists should particularly stress the dynamic aspect of working memory as a control center for decisions relevant to action, goal-oriented problem solving, associating new information with existing thought structures, and for shifting attention. Selective attention plays a central role in this, i.e., being able to concentrate on a new goal and to suppress former action motivations.

Possible Introduction by the Primary Therapist

Some time ago, we dealt with our memory, or more specifically speaking, with how we store texts, names, or numbers and retrieve them when required. Now we will look at memory from another perspective: How do we work with our memory? When reading a text for example, we rely on our memory to actively link separate sentences and words together so that we understand the text correctly. It also helps us associate information contained in the text with what we already know, i.e., what we have stored in our memory. We also work with our memory when we make a decision, solve a problem, or when we learn something new. We then have recourse to our experiences and connect new information with known information. When carrying out several tasks, we are forced to process various sources of information (stimuli) simultaneously. We are flooded with stimuli, yet we still have to concentrate. This is considerably different from our discussions about attentional performance during boring or monotonous work (understimulation). When we are overstimulated, it is important that we not allow ourselves to be too distracted (e.g., "I'm looking for a friend whom I'm supposed to meet at a concert. Many people are there, and the music is loud. If I concentrate too much on the music, I will probably not find my friend. It would be better to watch out for him and use his attributes to orient myself, e.g., hair color, height, or clothing. This means I have to focus my attention on a particular goal [selective attention] and not let myself be distracted.") Summing up, this means that we work with our memory very often.

To supplement the discussion, the group reads ► CD Information Sheet 30 ("Working actively with memory"). It differentiates between different functions of working memory. The primary therapist points out that, when working with memory, all the neurocognitive functions discussed up to this point are involved: speed of information processing, attention, memory, as well as reasoning and problem solving. Various behavioral experiments that can be done as a group are suitable for illustration:

Exercise: "Providing Information" The therapists select two participants. For the following role play, the latter are instructed to imagine that they leave the building together after the end of a group session. Outside they run into a tourist, who asks them for directions. However, the tourist is speaking another language. But the tourist's destination, a tourist attraction of the city, is pronounced approximately the same way in every language. The primary therapist could also choose a participant fluent in a foreign language to take the role of the tourist. Alternatively, the co-therapist can play the tourist. Various solution alternatives are discussed. The objective is to make it clear to both the active and passive participants that all of the aforementioned neurocognitive functions play a role in this situation.

Exercise: "Party Effect" The participants are asked to make conversation in groups of two or three about a current topic (hobbies, sport, etc.) with the instruction that they are not to let themselves be distracted. Once the therapists have ascertained that all participants could imagine the given situation, the less active therapist in the session (co-therapist) speaks a participant's name, first quietly and then increasingly loudly, until the addressed person responds. This question is then posed to the participant: "Why did you react to this?" Then the group discusses possible reasons ("A person knows her own name, heard it 100 times, etc."). Again, the aim of the exercise is to increase participants' awareness of the functions described above that are involved in the process. In addition, the exercise also addresses selective perception.

▪ Promoting Self-Perception in the Cognitive Target Area

Based on the introduction and the behavioral experiments, a first connection is now made to the participants' everyday lives.

? Examples of Key Questions

- In your everyday life (work, free time), have you ever experienced being exposed to (too) many stimuli, but you still have to concentrate on something?
- In what situations is it easier for you not to get distracted?
- Have you had everyday experiences in which you had to break away from what you were doing (e.g., watching TV) so you could concentrate on something completely different (e.g., making a phone call) or in which you were forced to carry our different activities at the same time (e.g., answering a phone call while cooking)?
- Have you ever had to quickly decide between different options while being afraid it could be wrong?
- Was that easy for you, or was it emotionally straining?
- What feelings did you have at the time?

The co-therapist notes down group contributions on the flip chart. In the process, the primary therapist asks the other participants each time a contribution is made whether they have also had the same experience in order to link the experiences of the group members. The therapists should encourage the participants to base their contributions on everyday experiences that are as concrete as possible. In conclusion, each participant fills out ► CD Worksheet 18 ("How well do I work with my memory in everyday life?").

▪ Case Vignettes

Following this, ► CD Vignettes 14 ("Recently at the bar") and 15 ("A busy day at work") are read as a group. After reading the vignettes, a group discussion connects the subject matter to the personal lives of the participants. Both vignettes focus on strain caused by overstimulation. ► CD Vignette 14 describes the effect of social overstimulation on concentration as well as strain caused by deviating from habit (Peter has to sit at an unaccustomed table in the middle of a bar).

? Examples of Key Questions

- Were there situations in which I felt uncomfortable and couldn't concentrate well because I was distracted by other people's noise and commotion?
- Has this happened often?
- In which situations?
- How did this make me feel?
- What did I do to better endure this situation?

Also the following general questions in order to promote self-reflection:

- Do I have difficulty when too much is happening around me?
- Am I more the kind of person who retreats from or even avoids such situation entirely?
- Or am I the kind of person who knows what to do in such situations?

The group then explores the individual, subjective experience of strengths and weaknesses in situations involving overstimulation. Once again, coping strategies are recorded for the time being to be discussed later in the compensation section.

► CD Vignette 15 ("A busy day at work") concentrates on the other hand on a typical work situation in which various tasks have to be finished on schedule. This means that Peter has to turn away from one activity to take care of a new one. This tends to be difficult for many participants. The didactic procedure is identical to that of ▶ CD Vignette 14. In addition, a role play can be acted out for illustration:

Role Play

The primary therapist selects two participants. Each receives several empty sheets of paper and a pen. The order of the fictitious boss is: "Draw regular hexagons and give them to your co-worker. For each hexagon you receive, shade in the six corners and write the first name of a group member in the center of the hexagon. Then give the hexagon back to your co-worker to be checked. At the end, there should be a paper with a hexagon, shadowed corners, and first name for each group member. Please do this as quickly and exactly as possible!"

As with ▶ CD Vignette 15, the group discusses where difficulties arose and how these could possibly be overcome in order to optimize the execution of the order the second time.

▪ Influential Factor: Overstimulation

With the help of the everyday experiences of the participants and interventions that have been carried out so far, potential disturbing influences which might affect working memory should be determined.

? Examples of Key Questions

- Have I experienced everyday situations in which I was not able to work with my memory optimally?
- How did this make me feel?
- Did it have something to do with the fact that I was surrounded by (many) people in this situation?
- What might have impaired work with memory in this situation?
- This impairment, was it triggered more by me – internally – or by my environment – externally?

For illustration and to review the activation graph introduced in Module A, the therapists now refer back to ▶ CD Information Sheet 2 ("Performance and mood"). In the interventions on vigilance in Module A, the focus was on the left side of the activation graph (low activation, understimulation). Now the right side is discussed (high activation, overstimulation). The point is to make a connection between overstimulation and reduced performance.

Please note that participant contributions from Module A on the topic of concentration loss from overstimulation and stress should also be taken into account here.

2.3.4.1.2 Compensation

In the compensation section, coping strategies for improving working memory are developed on the basis of the introductory section. The topic of internal or external overstimulation has already been introduced above. Participants often equate it in their daily lives with stress and emotional strain. Didactically speaking however, INT handles the topic of coping with stress and straining emotions in the following social-cognitive section of Module D.

The compensation section on working memory is organized into four basic areas:

- Concentration difficulties due to distraction and overstimulation
- Action rituals and cognitive flexibility when executing several actions
- Selective perception during overstimulation
- Concentration difficulties during a conversation

▪ Distraction and Overstimulation Caused by Sensory Overload

The intervention focuses initially on the ability to concentrate in situations of sensory overload. Concentration is understood as the precondition for being able to correctly perceive the demands of a concrete situation despite sensory overload and to act appropriately. Participants have already mentioned various concrete situations that are relevant to working memory in the introductory section, and these were noted down on the flip chart as usual by the therapists. These contributions should now be summarized and supplemented with additional concrete everyday situations of the participants. The group discusses the topic of concentration during sensory overload from the point of view of the possible negative effects of distraction and overstimulation.

? Examples of Key Questions

- Many people experience difficulties concentrating in various situations because they cannot shield themselves well from external or internal stimuli. Have you had everyday experiences of this?
- What is worse for you, internally (chains of thoughts, daydreams, etc.) or externally caused sensory overload (many people, noise, lights, smells, etc.)?
- In situations when e.g., the bus is overcrowded, everybody is speaking at once, the odor of sweat is in the air, and people got shaken by the bumpy ride, it is easy for us to be distracted. We are often overstimulated internally. Then we have the feeling that it's too much. Have you experienced comparable situations?
- What do you think and feel? How do you behave?

- What physical signals do you perceive in the process, like sweating, rapid heartbeat, difficulty breathing, restlessness, etc.?
- What do you do then? Do you tend to withdraw yourself from the situation or do you try to cope with it?
- For this reason, do you like to be with other people or do you prefer to be alone?

The questions above are discussed as a group. Again, arguments based on facts are preferable to assumptions. If there are differing opinions in particular, the primary therapist stresses that both the optimal level of internal activity and tolerance to stimuli can vary widely among individuals. Moreover, one's own tolerance to activity and stimuli can also vary depending on the situation and symptoms experienced. Supplementing the discussion, the group reads ► CD Worksheet 19 ("I was too distracted – I couldn't do anything!"). Participants provide individual answers to questions regarding sensory overload, subjective perception, and overstimulation and finally regarding coping strategies they have already applied. Participants' answers are then collected and discussed as a group. The objective is to promote participant self-reflection on the basis of situations they have experienced:

- with respect to their own reactions to overstimulation in the four areas
- with respect to coping strategies they have already tried out (below)

Reactions to Overstimulation

- **Cognitions/thinking:** thoughts such as "I can't take this anymore!", "I want to get out of here!", "Other people get on my nerves!", "Hopefully nobody notices that I can hardly stand this."
- **Emotions:** e.g., feelings of anxiety, rage, shame
- **Physical reactions:** e.g., sweating, palpitations, chest discomfort, tingling in the legs
- **Behavior:** restlessness, not being able to sit still, flight

Individually Applied Coping Strategies

These are compiled on the flip chart and evaluated in group discussion. As before, both resources and deficits in behavioral competency should be discussed equally.

Action Rituals

In the discussion of coping strategies with respect to sensory overload and resultant distraction, therapists take into account the action rituals often used by participants in their daily lives. Patients with schizophrenia have an increased need for security and coherence in their experience and behavior and for a feeling of control in everyday situations. Their action rituals are a sign of this need. Therapists should therefore avoid pulling the rug from under the participants' feet by taking an excessively change-oriented attitude, which would magnify their feelings of loss of control. The goal here is solely to promote insight. They should learn to balance the "benefits" (control, security) of action rituals with their potential "costs" (inflexibility, deviation from the norm, etc.). For illustration, ► CD Information Sheet 31 ("Costs and benefits of behavior change") is available on the accompanying ► CD-ROM. This information sheet presents a scale measuring the costs and benefits (advantages and disadvantages) of tried and tested behavioral and coping strategies compared with new. The costs and benefits of accustomed strategies are interchanged on the scale of the new strategies. The costs of accustomed strategies become the benefits of the new with an inverted sign.

Behavior	Benefits (Pros)	Costs (Cons)
Habit	....	....
New	....	....

Fig. 2.25 4-field diagram for promoting self-reflection as an orientation aid

To supplement this, the costs and benefits of accustomed action rituals and new approaches can be processed with the help of a 4-field diagram (Fig. 2.25). Costs/benefits or advantages/disadvantages can be referred here directly to the concrete situation and listed on the four fields. It is recommended that new behavior patterns that are appropriate to the situation and are potentially effective be filled in last in the "new-benefits" field. If the therapeutic process also aims at behavior change, the separate arguments written in the four fields can also be weighed, e.g., on a scale of 1–10, whereby 1 is unimportant and 10 is of maximum importance. The values of the individual fields are then added up and compared.

To bring the topic of action rituals closer to reality, we first have recourse to films:

For example, the film "As Good as it Gets" (with Jack Nicholson and Helen Hunt, USA 1997) has already proved effective in this context. The main character is a neurotic man with an obsessive personality. Associated compulsive rituals are the comedic focus of numerous scenes. As previously, the primary therapist only presents scenes of about 5-min length. The didactic approach to discussing film scenes has already been discussed in detail in Modules

B and C. Afterwards participants exchange experiences regarding personal rituals. The objective is to make them aware of the positive aspects of action rituals (security, feeling of control) as well as for negative consequences when they are used excessively (inflexibility, limitations, social consequences). This exercise requires a high level of group cohesion, trust, and stress resistance, since it addresses deeply rooted personal habits. Relinquishment of these habits can be associated with fear of losing control and damage to self-worth, especially among persons suffering from schizophrenia.

Adaptability Between Several Actions

Before the group returns to the topic of coping strategies for overstimulation in the following section, adaptability between different actions/activities is first discussed. This concerns the general difficulty of ending a current activity in order to move on to another activity. Those seeking structure and security often ritualize their activities, which is why it is usually difficult for them to switch between two or more activities in a flexible way that is appropriate to the situation. To connect with their everyday lives and to promote self-reflection, participants fill out ▶ CD Worksheet 20 ("Adaptability: being able to switch from one activity to another") on the enclosed ▶ CD-ROM. The aim is to support more discerning self-reflection on the part of the participants. The two final questions of ▶ CD Worksheet 20 regarding difficulties in adaptability (cognitive flexibility) serve to analyze these difficulties individually. The following group exercises are recommended for exemplifying adaptability.

Card-Sorting Exercise The primary therapist explains that adaptability also plays an important role in games, e.g., a rapid change of situations in a card game. For this purpose, the 96 cards (card-sorting exercise; ▶ CD Materials 2a–l) can be used. These were already employed in Module A on the subject of speed of information processing. While the aim then was to play the cards as quickly as possible, the point now is to make as few mistakes as possible. The basic rule – at least one feature of the card that was last played has to agree with the card being currently placed – is supplemented with the following additional rules:

1. Joker color: One card is randomly selected from the deck. Its color is the joker color from now on (blue, red, yellow, or green), which has the following characteristic: A card with the joker color can be placed without regard to the features of the previous card. So cards with the joker color can be played at any time.
2. Each participant receives 8–10 cards, which may be looked at, but not shown to other players.
3. The number of cards to be played: At least one card must be played per turn with a maximum of two cards. Then it is the next player's turn.
4. Sanctions: Whoever does not have a matching card that can be played has to take a substitute card; whoever makes an error has to also.
5. The first to play all of his or her cards wins. The group continues to play for the 2nd and 3rd places.

Matchstick Exercise This exercise is based on a scene from the film "Last year at Marienbad" (by Alain Resnais, France 1960), in which the following matchstick game appeared. Two players each receive a pile of matchsticks (at least 15). The rules are as follows: There are at least 15 matchsticks (or toothpicks) per pile. Two players play against each other. The first takes one, two, or three matchsticks from the pile. The other player repeats this. They take turns removing 1–3 matchsticks until no more are left in the pile. Whoever takes the last match loses. Some participants will soon notice that victory is well-nigh impossible if the opponent has to pull 1, 2, or 3 matchsticks from a pile of 5 (or 9). As with the card-sorting exercise described above, this exercise also places high demands on adaptability. Depending on the group composition, the therapists can play along in a tournament.

Further Exercises Various materials are available for individual exercises on the ▶ CD-ROM, which can be done here in parallel or in quick sequence in order to promote adaptability. ▶ CD Materials 14a–f each contain two pictures which differ in ten ways, which should be determined. ▶ CD Materials 15a–c contain word-search puzzles, in which given words must be found in a jumble of letters. ▶ CD Materials 16a–f contain easily solvable Sudoku puzzles of increasing difficulty. ▶ CD Materials 17a–c have texts with writing errors which must be identified. The exercises described on ▶ CD Materials 14–17 all challenge working memory in a larger sense. The objective is to have each participant work on at least two different exercises simultaneously. To this end, each participant receives 2–3 printed exercises. They are then instructed to switch from one exercise to the other in 3–5 min and then back again after the same time period. Therapists signal each change. This exercise is designed realistically and actively simulates shifting from one activity to the next. It is practiced repeatedly only in the following restitution section after the group has developed associated coping strategies.

Each of these exercises should be discussed in detail afterwards, and the resources and deficits experienced during the exercise compiled. The participants should become aware that they could compensate for their own functional deficits using coping strategies they have already developed. In addition, therapists can again refer to the topic of attention control in the concluding stress coping and emotion regulation section of this module.

Coping Strategies for Preventing Distraction During Overstimulation and for Improving Selective Attention

Individual coping strategies for reducing distractibility in overstimulating situations that were previously compiled are now repeated again in the group. Therapists should also return to ▶ CD Worksheet 19 ("I was too distracted – I couldn't do anything!"), on which the participants recorded their own coping strategies and everyday situations they experienced. To supplement this, ▶ CD Information Sheet 32 ("Strategies for avoiding distraction when performing actions") is available on the accompanying ▶ CD-ROM. This sheet lists easily applicable, action-oriented strategies referring to the two topics of "structuring action" and "choosing a helpful environment". In addition, the participants are asked to supplement both topics with their own strategies under the rubric of "further strategies". In the process, they also asses the coping strategies on the basis of concretely experienced, everyday situations to find if the strategies suit them or not. During the subsequent group discussion and evaluation of individual coping strategies for preventing distraction from sensory overload, the primary therapist again makes reference to the function of selective attention.

Example Formulation

We have now discussed possible strategies of protecting ourselves from too much distraction in situations in which a lot is happening and we may feel overly strained. While on the one hand we can protect ourselves from too much distraction, on the other we can also direct our attention consciously towards something interesting or towards a demanding situation. Are there situations in our daily life that force us to find particular information selectively from a wealth of information?

As a supplement to the coping strategies already collected (▶ CD Information Sheet 32 "Strategies for avoiding distraction when performing actions"), the group also develops strategies for improving selective attention and reducing distractibility with the help of ▶ CD Information Sheet 33 ("Focusing concentration"). Further strategies volunteered by participants during discussion should be noted on ▶ CD Information Sheet 33. The strategies should be discussed in using as many everyday examples as possible. Discussion focuses on experiencing and dealing with stress-inducing situations. Both in vivo exercises outside the therapy setting and independent exercises help the participants apply the coping strategies in similar situations.

The following group exercise can be carried out to give the participants their first experiences with compensating impairments in selective perception:

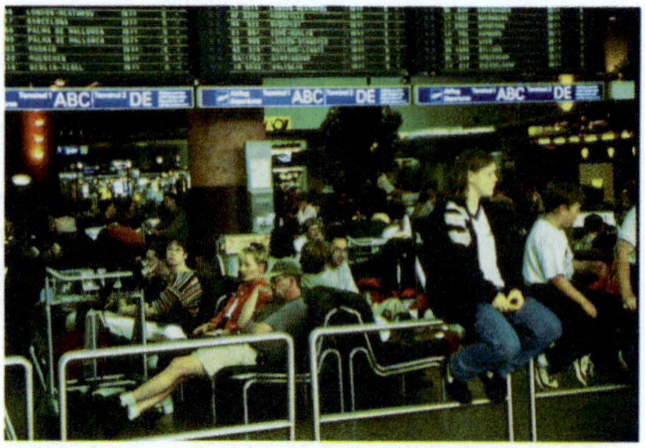

◘ **Fig. 2.26** Pictures on selective perception (Photos: V. Roder, with kind permission)

Selective Perception with Pictures Along with ▶ CD e-Materials 9 (e9a–h: "Picture series: selective perception") a picture series with a high level of complexity is also available (◘ Fig. 2.26). This series will be worked on more than once in the following restitution section. At this point, only one or two pictures should be selected, however. There are two versions of the exercise for the 8 pictures: In version 1, one picture is presented for 30 s and then described by the whole group with the help of stored information. In version 2, the group looks for a target stimulus on the presented image (Examples of target stimuli are listed on slide 9. We will proceed here only with variant 2.)

Didactic Procedure

1. To prepare for the exercise, the group reviews the coping strategies listed on ▶ CD Information Sheets 32 and 33.
2. The exercise begins with the presentation of a selected picture (▶ CD e-Materials 9a–h). The scene depicted on it should first be objectively and succinctly described (see ▶ Sect. 2.3.2.2).
3. In the next step, the primary therapist poses specific questions about cue stimuli. ◘ Figure 2.26 provides an example of possible questions about target stimuli: "I need to post a letter. Can you tell me where I can find a post office?", "I'm looking for my brother. He's wearing a striped shirt. Have you seen him?", "I'm thirsty. Where can I get something to drink?", etc.
4. When answering each question, the group discusses which strategies were helpful for finding the target stimulus.
5. The final step is to establish a connection to the participants' personal experience. Possible key questions include: "Have I experienced these or similar situations?", "What kinds of feelings do such situations trigger in me?", "How do I cope with that?" The focus of the intervention is on adaptive coping strategies in

stress-inducing situations. These will be discussed in more detail in conclusion within the intervention section on coping with stress and emotion regulation.

▪ Coping Strategies for Preventing Distraction During a Conversation

At the conclusion of the compensation section, the group focuses on distractibility during conversation. This is often experienced as particularly stress-inducing and straining. The first goal is to identify what the individual stress factors in a conversation are. As usual, it is important that existing resources are reinforced and compiled contributions are recorded in writing.

? Examples of Key Questions

- Sometimes we find it difficult to follow a conversation. What are the reasons for this?
- What are possible triggers for our own distraction?
- In what concrete situations and under what conditions do we usually find it easier or harder to concentrate on a conversation?
- Are there persons with whom it is easier or harder to have a conversation? What differentiates them from others?

The next step is to compare and record participants' personal experiences with applying their own strategies.

- How can I improve my power of concentration during conversation?

These are then supplemented with the coping strategies found on ▶ CD Information Sheet 34 ("Distractibility during conversation"). Any additional coping strategies developed during group discussion should be added individually by the participants onto ▶ CD Information Sheet 34. At the end, each participant should have available an individual repertoire of different coping strategies.

To give the participants the chance to experience individualized coping strategies and their consequences, role plays of varying degrees of difficulty are suitable for the group context. Role plays can be used, for example, to realistically simulate concrete everyday situations. Possible examples include the following:

Restaurant Visit The participants sit at a large table and are asked to split in twos and make conversation with each other. All the pairs carry out conversations simultaneously. If there are an uneven number of participants, the co-therapist takes part in the exercise as well. Topics of conversation should include present day experiences made by both conversation partners: the way to the group room, further plans for the evening, etc. The current listeners within the conversation pairs attempt to fill gaps in the partner's schedule by asking specific questions. The roles are then exchanged and the listener becomes the interviewee. Participants should be able to give an account that is as detailed as possible of the partner's experiences that day after the role play. The level of difficulty can be varied. For example, a radio can be played in the background. It is advantageous to perform this role play directly after working on ▶ CD Information Sheet 34. If required, the strategies for improving attention described on it should be reviewed once again. Crucial strategies in this context include "eye contact", "repetition", and "questions". These are examples of possible strategies in case the first strategy of "reducing distraction" is not possible. The exercise should not go on any longer than 10 min. A round of feedback follows.

Dinner with Roommates The therapists select two participants. They are instructed to have a conversation involving a question-answer situation, which first has to be defined. One of these participants is asked to pose a concrete question to the conversation partner (e.g., a calculation task, questions about sport events). The conversation partner's task is to answer the question. Before carrying out the role play, the rest of the group members need to be given their side roles. While simulating a common dinner at a shared apartment, they should talk about such and such, ask to pass the bread, coffee, or butter, and even simulate the act of eating by smacking their lips. After a brief rehearsal with the supporting actors, the role play starts and both of the target participants begin their question-answer game. The primary strategy to be applied here is "asserting oneself over others for a short time" on ▶ CD Information Sheet 34. This refers to drawing the attention of others to one self briefly in order to concentrate on the question ("Please be quiet for a moment. I want to answer this question, and then you can continue talking"). This exercise, which tends to be straining for many participants, requires an extensive feedback session. If the role play is repeated, it can be helpful for the participants to fill out ▶ CD Worksheet 4 ("My helpful strategies for…") beforehand in order to clearly define and internalize the coping strategies to be applied. In principle, most of the concrete, everyday situations brought up by the participants can be simulated in a role play.

2.3.4.1.3 Restitution

The restitution section combines group exercises, some of which were already introduced and described in the compensation section, and computer-based exercises. Before each exercise, the participants receive ▶ CD Worksheet 4 ("My helpful strategies for…") and fill it out individually.

The following will first describe the group exercises and then the computer-based exercises.

2

Group Exercises

Some of the group exercises were already done in the compensation section. The following group exercises are now carried out repeatedly using the available materials.

Cognitive Flexibility Card-sorting exercise (▶ CD Materials 2a–l): the game rules were described in the compensation section. Different possibilities of variation can be made use of. For example, a higher number of cards to be played (including penalty cards) gradually increases the level of difficulty. The number of joker colors (two instead of one) can also be varied. Group dynamics can be promoted didactically by forming teams, within which cards can be exchanged.

Cognitive Flexibility and Learning Strategy Matchstick exercise (scene from the film "Last year at Marienbad" by Alain Resnais, Frankreich 1960): The level of difficulty depends on the number of matchsticks. Depending on group cohesion, a tournament among both participants and therapists is possible.

Action Change (Performing Several Tasks Simultaneously ▶ CD Materials 14–17) This series of exercises, introduced in the compensation section, should be repeated at this point so that the participants can habituate "letting go of one activity and moving on to another activity". The level of strain is increased with the number of individual activities (differences between two pictures, word-search puzzle, Sudoku, text with writing errors) as well as the intervals of time available.

Selective Perception Picture series (▶ CD e-Materials 9a–h): There are two versions of this picture-based exercise. Version 2 has already been described in the compensation section.

The following additional group exercises are provided:

Cognitive Flexibility IPT card-sorting exercise (▶ CD Materials 1): The same cards that were already used in Modules A–C are used here in a modified exercise. As before, each participant (and the therapists) receives 6–8 cards, which are placed face-up on the table. One participant is asked to note down the characteristics of one or two cards on a sheet of paper without the others seeing the notes. Now participants take turns asking about the characteristics of the target cards. Only yes or no answers are allowed.

Selective Perception Picture series (▶ CD e-Materials 9a–h), version 1: Version 1 places high demands on the participants, since it relates to all the cognitive intervention areas of Modules A–C. The group members should first try committing the picture to memory (overall impression and details).

1. A selected picture is projected for 30 s and then disappears again.
2. The group is now instructed to described the picture that was shown from memory: "What kind of situation was depicted?", "What were some important details?", "Where were these details on the picture?" etc. The co-therapist either writes or draws the participants' contributions on the flip chart.
3. Afterwards, the sketch or notes are compared with the initial image. Didactically speaking, it is recommended that the therapists follow a highly structured procedure.

Distractibility in Conversation (Role Play) Other concrete situations are simulated in role plays. On the one hand, this promotes certainty in the use of cognitive compensation strategies in social contexts. On the other hand, the role plays also serve as a preparation for individual exercises (homework) and in vivo exercises.

Test-Psychological Exercise on Working Memory For this exercise, lists with several series of numbers, letters, and words are available on the enclosed ▶ CD-ROM (▶ CD Materials 18a–b, exercises a–j). The co-therapist reads out loud a series of items from two categories (e.g., numbers and letters). The participants are then asked to recall these items from memory in a predetermined order and to combine them into categories (e.g., give first the letters in alphabetical order and then in the numbers in increasing order). This exercise can be done in two versions:

- Participants solve the task together as a group. They discuss which items were recalled correctly and which sequence matches the task at hand. The co-therapist then records their results on the flip chart.
- In addition, each participant solves the task individually. For this, each receives a pen and a sheet of paper. The individual solutions should then be compiled and compared.

Computer-Based Exercises

Didactically, the CogPack exercises are implemented in the same manner as in Modules A–C. The following CogPack exercises are available:

SEARCH This typical exercise on selective perception consists of 18 sub-exercises. Both the correctness and speed of the solutions are measured. In the first three sub-exercises a–c (easy, medium, hard), a target stimulus (number) must be identified. In sub-exercises d–h (the Ninth), the missing number in the series of 1 to 9 must be identified.

The sub-exercises i–n (double), one number is shown twice in the same number series. In the rest of the sub-exercises o–r (double, triple, adaptive) on the other hand, letters have to be identified that appear more than once in a series. All sub-exercises of SEARCH are recommendable.

CONNECT In this exercise, different points have to be connected according to a given order. The points consist of figures or letters. Eight sub-exercises are included (a–h).

MONEY The 20 sub-exercises (q-t) all refer to the use of coins and bills. Their level of difficulty can be varied.

COLORS&LABELS This classic interference and selective perception exercise consists of nine sub-exercises (a-i). In each, color/label interferences or a "missing" or "false" color has to be identified.

INTERFERENCE This exercise consists of two sub-exercises (a–b). In sub-exercise a, color/label interferences should be identified. In sub-exercise b, the goal is to identify target stimuli from a group of distracting and target stimuli as quickly as possible.

LINESEGMENTS In a total of 20 sub-exercises, the objective is to divide a line into 2,3,4, or 5 parts of equal size. In the last three sub-exercises (r–q), the starting line must be divided into various parts of equal size. The level of difficulty increases from exercise a to exercise t.

PIESEGMENTS This exercise consists of three sub-exercises (a–c). Like the exercise LINESEGMENTS, the objective is to cut a pie into a given number of pieces of equal size. The level of difficulty increases from exercise a to exercise c.

QUANTITY In two sub-exercises a–b (quick, no distraction; slow, distraction), target stimuli are displayed and their quantity must be estimated after being hidden.

GEOMETRY Of the seven sub-exercises (a–g), only sub-exercise a (polyhedrons) is recommendable. In it, the features of three-dimensional polygons must be determined. This exercise is also highly suitable for the individual advancement of especially capable participants.

SEQUENCE This exercise consists of a total of 12 series of numbers or letters that have to be continued. Behind each sequence is a strategy or simple (mathematical) operation of how the sequence is built. The requirement profile of this exercise is relatively high. Accordingly, this exercise should be utilized to promote especially capable participants on an individual basis.

The following exercises were already used and described in Module B (verbal and visual memory) and can be repeated here: NEWorNOT, OntheRoad, READING, and GEOGRAPHY.

As in Modules A–C, group and computer exercises are preformed in alternation. After each block of exercises, both difficulties and successes are collected and analyzed. With the help of ▶ CD Information Sheets 30–34 as well as ▶ CD Worksheets 4, 19–20, the group discusses the personal benefits and difficulties of their application.

Here too, the participants check over and correct the assessments they initially made of their own performance ("How well do I work with my memory in everyday life?").

2.3.4.1.4 In Vivo Exercises and Independent Exercises

In conclusion, in vivo exercises are carried out, and participants' readiness to perform independent tasks is promoted. The independent exercises take into account the examples volunteered by the participants of difficulties and resources they have experienced in their everyday lives. The personal notes of the participants on ▶ CD Worksheets 19–20 and the everyday situations they described serve as a foundation for this. In order to prepare for the independent exercise, each member of the group first fills out ▶ CD Worksheet 5 ("Independent exercise"). The particular steps are described in detail in Module B. Examples of possible tasks in the area of working memory include:

- Carrying on a conversation or reading a newspaper during a bus ride, thereby applying learned coping strategies against distraction during overstimulation.
- Planning and executing a shopping excursion: making shopping lists and going shopping at a department store or supermarket.
- Structuring actions, e.g., finding the planned route in the hustle of the city.
- Planning on reading something specific and considering when and where this would be best done. Only the result counts!
- Making an appointment with someone at a well-known, bustling meeting place.
- Participating and asserting oneself in a conversation at a restaurant or during dinner with roommates at an apartment or with family.

In addition to independent exercises, in vivo exercises with the group can be performed using the above examples. The level of strain triggered by the target situation should initially be kept as low as possible and then gradually increased. Strain levels are generally highest during social interactions.

Example

The INT group is planning an excursion into town. The objective is to take a stroll through the largest department store in town and to inquire casually about the wares. Each participant makes a list of 2–5 items (▶ CD Worksheet 5) that are of personal interest. They then compare their lists in order to find potential correspondences. The group categorizes the target wares and assigns them to corresponding departments of the store (e.g., ladies/menswear, sports goods, household, etc.). Then subgroups are assembled, consisting of participants who wish to go together to the various departments. In addition, each participant considers what difficulties they anticipate and how these are to be overcome (▶ CD Worksheet 5). Finally, the INT group goes into town with the therapist team. Proceeding from a common meeting point, the subgroups look for their predetermined departments. Every in vivo exercise concludes with a discussion immediately afterwards or at the start of the next session.

2.3.4.2 Social-Cognitive Intervention Area: Social Attributions and Emotion Regulation

Module D: Social-Cognitive Intervention Area: Social Attributions and Emotion Regulation

1. Introduction
   - Introduction: attributions
     - Definition: causal attribution and conclusions; internal and external causal attribution
     - Self-perception in the target area
     - Resource-oriented individual profile in the target area
     - Connection to self and everyday life Case Vignette
     - Influential factors
   - Introduction: emotion regulation
     - Vulnerability and stress
     - Controlling emotions
     - Self-perception in the target area
     - Connection to self and everyday life Case vignette
2. Compensation
   - Examining one's own attributions and their consequences
   - Reattribution: developing alternative causal attributions
   - Strategies for reducing stress and regulating emotion
3. Restitution
   - Habituation of learned coping strategies in repeated group exercises: causal attribution in four stages using various materials, coping with stress and regulating emotion
4. In vivo exercises and independent exercises
   - Transfer of individualized coping strategies to concrete, everyday situations
   - Integrating all learned compensation strategies of the four modules into planned, concrete everyday situations

Tips

- Infrastructure: group therapy room, flip chart, projector
- Therapy materials: ▶ CD Information Sheets 35–42, ▶ CD Worksheets 4–5, 21–24, ▶ CD Vignettes 16–17, ▶ CD Materials 19–21, ▶ CD e-Materials 10, commercial videos
- Didactics: structured group discussion and role plays

2.3.4.2.1 Introductory Sessions

2.3.4.2.1.1 Introduction: Attribution

▪ Definition of the Target Area

In the final section of Module D, the interventions initially focus on social attributions and then on emotion regulation. According to the MATRICS initiative (Green et al. 2005), social attributions are defined as individual causal explanations for particular experiences of success or failure. They contribute to the understanding of social situations and events. This function, also designated as causal attribution in social and cognition psychology, reflects the human tendency to wish to get to the bottom of what causes observable events. Attributions thus have a structuring and orienting function. They also attempt to make events predictable. This depends on whether the person concerned views the cause of the event as stemming from himself or herself (internally) or from others/the environment (externally). It also depends on whether the person experiences the situation as variable (random) or stable (the same will occur in future), as controllable or noncontrollable. In other words, attributions are automatic assessment processes within our working memory.

In schizophrenia research, attributions are also investigated as meta-cognitive influences forming the basis of positive symptoms. These are treated, especially in English-speaking countries, by means of cognitive therapy (Cognitive Behavior Therapy for Psychosis, CBTp).

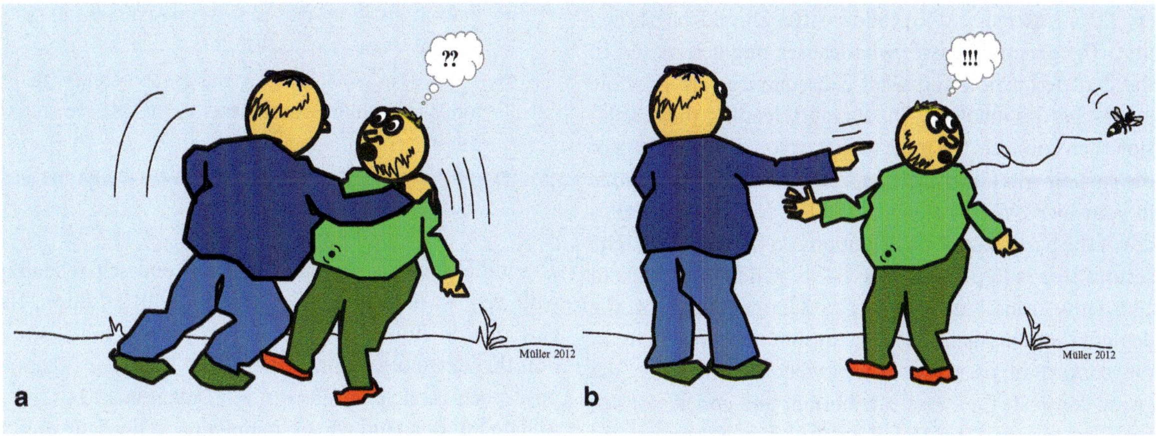

■ **Fig. 2.27** (**a, b**) Attribution. Picture (**a**) Why is the man in the blue sweater acting that way towards Peter? How does Peter react to this? Picture (**b**) Why did the man in the blue sweater act that way towards Peter? How is Peter reacting now?

In contrast to this, INT defines attributions as a social-cognitive function or as a cognitive "symptom" (deficit). The goal is that the participants acquire coping strategies that enable them to implement this social-cognitive function more appropriately to the situation and that errors in attribution are reduced, thereby stabilizing patients' self-worth in social situations. However, should some of the participants exhibit prominently persisting positive symptoms, they should be referred to an accompanying CBTp in a one-on-one setting as well as to an optimization of the pharmacotherapeutic intervention.

As in previous intervention units, the concept of social attributions, abstract for most participants, is defined. The concept of attribution is replaced with the more common concepts of "drawing conclusions" and "ascribing causes". In the introduction, the therapists should make connections to previous treatment topics as before.

Introduction Example

We have already dealt with how we can better cope with sensory overload in social situations without being too distracted. We saw that stimuli that distract us can be caused internally or externally. We will now focus more on what kinds of internal distraction sometimes prevent us from behaving successfully when interacting with others. We have already talked about how it is important in conversation to distinguish between fact and assumption and how we can better recognize the feelings of others – how we can guess what the other person might be thinking. But when something particular happens in our daily lives, this can make us insecure, for example when someone looks at or addresses us in a certain way. It is natural for us to wish to orient ourselves. We want to know what is happening and why. So we tend automatically to ascribe a cause to every event and to draw a conclusion from this. We will now take a closer look at ascribing causes and drawing conclusions. The cause I assign to an event and the conclusion I draw from this also affects my condition and has consequences for my behavior. When I am mistaken, and it turns out later that I ascribed a false cause to an event and thus drew the wrong conclusions, highly adverse consequences can result and put unnecessarily strain on others and me.

The following behavioral experiment serves to illustrate false causal attribution and conclusion:

Behavioral Experiment The primary therapist announces a short behavioral exercise. The co-therapists then stares in the direction of a (previously undetermined and unprepared) participant seated at least 3–4 m away. The co-therapist's gaze is not aimed at the target's eyes however, but on an object just past that person's left or right ear (e.g., the wall or the participant sitting just behind). In the meantime, the primary therapist asks the target person (who is probably somewhat surprised), whether she has noticed that the co-therapist is staring at her? Why is the co-therapist doing this? What is the target person thinking and feeling in the process? Only after the target has given brief answer to these questions with the help of other group members does the primary therapist ask whether the co-therapist actually looked at the target in the eyes. Where else might the co-therapist been looking? And would the co-therapist have even noticed whether the target participant had changed her viewing direction without moving her head? The objective is to make the influence of facts and assumptions on attributions clear and to indicate the possible consequences of false attributions.

As additional introduction to the topic of false attributions and the often emotionally stressful consequences, the comics shown in ■ Fig. 2.27a, b can be presented to the group – also available on the enclosed ► CD-ROM as slides

2

(▶ CD e-Materials 10a–b). Slide e-10a should be shown first. The group discusses what causes might have led to the depicted action and what consequences are possible for the parties involved. The therapist leading the discussion then connects the topic to the personal experiences of the participants ("Have you experienced similar situations in your lives? What happened?"). The co-therapist writes down the participants' contributions on the flip chart. The second step is to present slide e-10b, which now leads to alternative causal attributions and conclusions of the depicted action. Again, the content should be dealt with in the context of participants' everyday lives. Finally, the group contrasts the causal attributions and conclusions of both images (▶ CD e-Materials 10a–b) as observers and discusses the strains and emotions triggered (e.g., surprise, fear, relief, thankfulness). In addition, the quality of the triggered feelings should be determined (e.g., fear of violence in slide e10a vs. fear of being stung by a hornet in slide e-10b).

▪ Internal and External Attributions

Proceeding on the basis of the above intervention and the everyday experiences compiled, the objective now is to clarify the function of attributions in everyday experience. Participants should first learn to distinguish between internal causal attribution (derived from oneself) and external causal attribution (ascribed to other people or the situation). For this purpose, the group now reads ▶ CD Information Sheet 35 ("Is it my fault or someone else's? Internal vs. external causes") on the enclosed ▶ CD-ROM. The group also discusses the conclusions and consequences associated with causal attributions. As always, the primary therapist should motivate the participants to substantiate their contributions with concretely experienced situations from their everyday lives whenever possible.

▪ Promoting Self-Perception in the Cognitive Target Area

INT strives to link therapy content with participants' everyday lives in order to encourage self-perception in the target area. In the interventions described above, the participants have usually already volunteered some examples. These should now be supplemented and categorized as internal or external causal attribution (▶ CD Information Sheet 35).

? Possible Key Questions for Group Discussion

- We have already collected various everyday situations on the flip chart. Can these be assigned either to internal or external causal attribution?
- In what situations do you tend to ascribe the cause of a social event to others?
- In what situations do you tend to ascribe the cause of a social event to yourself?
- These days, would you say you are someone who tends to attribute everything to yourself or to others?
- Is the way you assign causes different in moments of success and of failure?

The initial focus is on self-perception and self-reflection with respect to one's own attributions. In addition, the participants should assess how appropriately to the situation they attribute event in their daily lives. For this purpose, each participant fills out ▶ CD Worksheet 21 ("How well do I understand what is happening in my daily life?"), which is discussed analogously to the method described above.

▪ Case Vignette

One case vignette is available on the subject of attribution on the accompanying ▶ CD-ROM (▶ CD Vignette 16: "A truly successful day?"). The vignette is read section-by-section as described above. Three causal attributions and conclusions are contained in it:

- Bruno's qualification interview,
- Peter's qualification interview, and
- Peter's date with Manuela.

The group discusses what consequences the attributions described in the vignette yield and how the protagonists feel as a result. The participants are again asked whether they have had similar experiences in their everyday lives. As usual, the co-therapist makes a written record of all contributions.

▪ Factors That Influence Attribution

Until now, individual and situational conditions that can influence attribution in a certain social situation were excluded. Following up on the previous interventions, the aim now is to direct participants' attention to identifying possible influential factors. Previous participant contributions concerning how they can change their own causal attribution should now be assimilated. The objective is to support participants in reflecting on differences in their own attributions in various situations.

? Examples of Key Questions

- Do you always ascribe events to causes in the same way, assigning responsibility usually to yourself or usually to others?
- If not, what influences you to assign responsibility sometimes to yourself and at other times to others?
- Does it have more to do with you, with others, or with the situation?

- Does it make a difference whether you are directly affected by the event or can witness it as a neutral observer?
- What are the differences?
- Can you describe concrete experiences of this?

In the following longer group discussions, therapists should pay special attention to how strongly the influential factors mentioned by participants are influenced by their persisting positive symptoms. If the influence of delusional ideas is very great or if a participant otherwise requires it, one-on-one sessions should also be offered. Depending on the capacity of the therapists, accompanying one-on-one talks can also refer the participant concerned to his or her psychotherapist or specialist for further guidance on the topic. Generally speaking, the procedure should remain transparent, and therapists should make the distinction between attribution as a cognitive function and as an indication of symptoms. The latter is not a direct intervention goal.

▶ CD Information Sheet 36 ("What can influence me in ascribing causes?") is read and discussed as a supplement to the influential factors already compiled and recorded. On it, the following dimensions of attribution are summarized:

- ascribing the causes of an event to ourselves or to others,
- experiencing causes as stable or variable,
- experiencing causes as controllable or non-controllable, and
- casual attribution as affected by one's current state of stress.

Finally, participants also have the opportunity to add other dimensions of attribution to ▶ CD Information Sheet 36, e.g., the influential factors learned in Modules A–C such as alertness, quality of sleep, mood, or attentional performance.

The dimensions of attribution are discussed using concrete examples provided by the group members or using model examples presented by the therapists. The goal is to demonstrate various conclusions depending on the attribution dimension as well as resultant emotional consequences (fear, anger, surprise, pleasure, pride, etc.) and behavioral consequences (flight and withdrawal, aggression, opening up to the other person, etc.). Combinations of attribution dimensions are also possible (stably uncontrollable vs. variably uncontrollable, etc.). During these group discussions, some participants might reach the limits of their processing capacity. Therapists can counter this by increasing the amount of conversational structure and by reducing the information's level of difficulty.

2.3.4.2.1.2 Introduction: Emotion Regulation

In direct continuation of the influence of stress and emotional strain on attribution style, introduced in the last section (▶ CD Information Sheet 36), the following section will now discuss emotion regulation for the first time. This final topic of INT is organized into two parts: First the experience of stress is discussed, followed by emotion regulation itself. Participants have made various contributions to these topics in previous interventions, which were recorded and put aside. The therapists should now return to these and reintroduce them at the appropriate time. The primary therapist provides a brief introduction to the influence of stress and straining emotions on cognitive performance.

Introduction Example

We have already dealt with the topic of ascribing causes to events and associated conclusions and consequences for one's own condition and behavior. This can trigger feelings, but can also be influenced by feelings in turn. We also learned that too many stimuli could result in stress. We will now discuss how stress and associated feelings – often negative – can adversely affect our performance in reasoning. Together we will then discuss strategies for coping with stress and for regulating negative feelings.

▪ Vulnerability and Stress

In order to promote self-reflection about participants' own experiences of stress, a reduced vulnerability/stress model is now introduced. This functions at the same time as a didactic basis for developing stress-coping strategies in the following compensation section. Based on a psychoeducational approach developed by our team (Roder et al. 2008b), ▶ CD Information Sheet 37 ("Vulnerability and stress") on the enclosed ▶ CD-ROM provides a vulnerability/stress model. Therapists should take heed that participants do not represent vulnerability as a fixed construct but rather as a relatively stable disposition. The objective for the time being is to explain the relationship between vulnerability and stress in symptom development. It should also be pointed out that stress can have both internal and external causes.

▪ Controlling Emotions

At the conclusion of Module D, the group learns and practices coping strategies for improving the regulation of emotions. Emotion regulation encompasses processes with which persons influence what emotions they have at a certain time and how they experience and express these emotions (Groß and Thompson 2007). Accordingly, this topic intersects with the construct of coping previously discussed. Both have the goal of reducing negative emotional states. Yet coping also includes non-emotional actions, which serve to achieve non-emotional goals. On the other hand, emotion-regulatory goals and actions are always geared towards emotions. Moreover, emotion-regulatory processes not only strive to reduce negative emotions, but also to reinforce or maintain positive emotions (Groß and Thompson 2007). The aim of this intervention unit is thus to enable the participants to control the quality and intensity of their feelings independently and thereby to establish an adaptive emotional state.

In the social-cognitive section of Module A, the participants developed an understanding of the function of the most crucial categorical emotions. It became clear to them that emotions are associated with certain automatic or learned behavioral tendencies aimed at simplifying interactions with the environment and ordering them efficiently. Emotions can also become too intense, too prolonged, or too inappropriate to the situation, resulting in the need for regulation. The following is a possible introduction to the topic of emotion regulation:

Introduction Example

We have already discussed extensively how we can recognize emotions in other people. In the process, we also noticed that emotions are actually helpful for us. For example, if we experience intense fear, this warns us about a dangerous situation. But emotions can also strain us. This is the case when they are too intense, last too long, and/or don't fit the situation. For example, persons who have arachnophobia often experience intense and prolonged fear, even if the spider is actually harmless. So in this session we will deal with how we can better control our emotions so we can experience fewer negative and more positive emotions. This ability is also called emotion regulation.

This information is summarized for the participants on ► CD Information Sheet 38.

▪ Promoting Self-Perception in the Cognitive Target Area

The following section is concerned with promoting participant self-reflection with respect to personal experiences of stress and emotion in everyday life. Everyday examples already mentioned by participants should be reviewed and additional experiences should be elicited for group discussion.

Examples of Key Questions

- Do you often experience stress in everyday life? Are there situation in which this happens frequently and others in which it hardly ever happens?
- Have you already thought about why this is the case? Are there certain stress triggers?
- Do you avoid stress or can you cope with stress well?
- In what situations do you tend to experience strong feelings? Do you experience severe stress in these situations?
- Do you find feeling helpful or aggravating and threatening?
- What is a good feeling for you? A bad feeling?
- Can you influence your own feelings?

The group discusses coping with stress and feelings, and participant comments are written down. Coping strategies are developed in the following compensation section. For now, the focus is on self-perception. In addition, each participant fills out ► CD Worksheet 22 ("How well can I cope with stress? How well can I control my feelings?"), which is discussed according to the method described above.

▪ Case Vignette

One case vignette is available for this intervention area on the accompanying ► CD-ROM (► CD Vignette 17: "This time everything went well!"). The first part of the vignette describes a successful experience of coping with stress. The second part depicts an example of emotion regulation that is appropriate to the situation. The vignette has two parts. Peter first experiences a stress-inducing situation (bus ride with sensory overload) and then an affectively straining situation (refused entry at a dance club). However, he masters both situations well. The vignette is read, in accordance with the aforementioned procedure, paragraph-by-paragraph. This is followed by making an initial connection to participants' own everyday experiences with coping with stress and emotional strain.

Examples of Key Questions

- How does Peter deal with the stress he experiences in the crowded bus? How does he influence his negative emotions, like anxiety and anger, before entering the dance club?
- Have you had personal experiences of such situations? How do you behave in such situations?
- How often and in what situations do you experience stress? How do you deal with it?
- What feelings are triggered in the process?
- How long do (straining) feelings last? How do you deal with them?
- Is your ability to think and to reason impaired by this?

2.3.4.2.2 Compensation

The group now develops coping strategies for the three topics discussed in the introductory section: attribution, stress, and emotion regulation. These should then be individualized for each participant. Didactically, these three topics are handled separately. This section begins with compensation strategies concerned with attribution style, followed by stress-coping strategies, and finally by strategies for improving emotion regulation.

▪ Examining One's Own Attributions and Their Consequences

The first item of importance is to direct the participants' focus on these evaluation processes, which are activated often and function automatically. In other words, the participant's own process of attribution and resultant conclusions should be constantly borne in mind. For this purpose, therapists can turn back to ▶ CD Information Sheets 35–36, which list various dimensions of causal attribution. In order to give participants the more opportunity to analyze their own causal attributions and conclusions in a concrete situation, it is recommended to carry out a group exercise in the form of a role play.

▪▪ Role Play

A concrete situation described by a participant in the introductory section will be simulated here as a role play. Alternatively, an example situation involving attribution included on the enclosed ▶ CD-ROM can serve as the basis for a role play (▶ CD Materials 19–21), such as the following statement: "When Peter went to the laundry room of his apartment block last week, he ran into his new neighbor. But he couldn't remember her name. When he returned to the laundry room today, he met the new neighbor again." Two participants under the guidance of the primary therapist briefly act out this situation according to the usual procedure. Then the analysis begins: The specific features of the situation should be summarized (laundry room, meeting the neighbor with the unknown name twice). After this, the participant in the role of Peter is asked for his spontaneous explanation (hypothesis) for meeting the same neighbor more than once. Then the rest of the group and finally the person in the role of the neighbor are asked the same (e.g., "Meeting twice was just a coincidence!" vs. "The neighbor waited for Peter because she wants to monitor him!"). The participants concerned are then asked what conclusions they draw from their explanations and what this could mean for them (e.g., "I don't have to worry about it, it was just a coincidence!" vs. "I knew it all along – I should be more careful in future!"). Finally, they are asked what consequences this has for their feelings, thoughts, physical reactions, and behavioral reactions.

This didactic procedure is also presented on ▶ CD Worksheet 23 ("Analyzing spontaneous causal attributions"). Several copies are distributed to the participants, because, in the following exercises, participants should become aware of and analyze their own spontaneous attributions before developing alternative attributions. Special attention should be paid to emotional reactions, because they will be the subject of the final section concerning emotion regulation.

▪ Reattribution

Once the participants have analyzed their own spontaneous attributions as well as ensuing conclusions and reactions in the example situations, the task now is to judge appropriateness in the concrete situation. If the appropriateness of a spontaneous attribution is questionable, alternative ways of explaining what has happened should be pursued. But first the level of strain caused by spontaneous causal attributions should be addressed. If one's individual attribution style yields psychological strain, reattribution should relieve that strain in a way that is immediately discernible to the person concerned. This also increases the willingness to change ("If I didn't relate everything back to myself, I would be doing better!"). On the other hand, if the individual attribution style primarily serves to maintain one's own self-concept ("I knew it all along that other people are following me!"), willingness to change will be quite low, and resistance can be expected. In this case, the aim of INT is to motivate the persons concerned to reflect on this in further-reaching conversations with their own individual therapists.

The initial objective is to establish a connection to participants' everyday experiences of their own individual attribution styles. Therapists should clarify whether and with what experiences the participants have questioned their own causal attributions in concrete situations.

? Examples of Key Questions

- Have you have had the experience that your spontaneous assumptions about and explanations of a situation weren't accurate?
- What did you do then?
- Did you try to find new explanations?
- What helped you do this?
- Are there certain strategies and tricks you could use?

As usual, the co-therapist makes a written record of all contributions. Depending on the level of group cohesion, the number of participant contributions may be low because of the amount of strain associated with the topic. If this is the case, therapists can have recourse to the aforementioned example situations on the ▶ CD-ROM as alternative or supplement models (▶ CD Materials 19–21). Finally, the group reads and discusses ▶ CD Information Sheet 39 ("Strategies for examining our own spontaneous causal attribution"). This contains strategies for monitoring and (if necessary) modifying one's own spontaneous assumptions regarding the cause of an event. Participants should learn to examine their spontaneous conclusions with the help of facts and to find alternative ways of

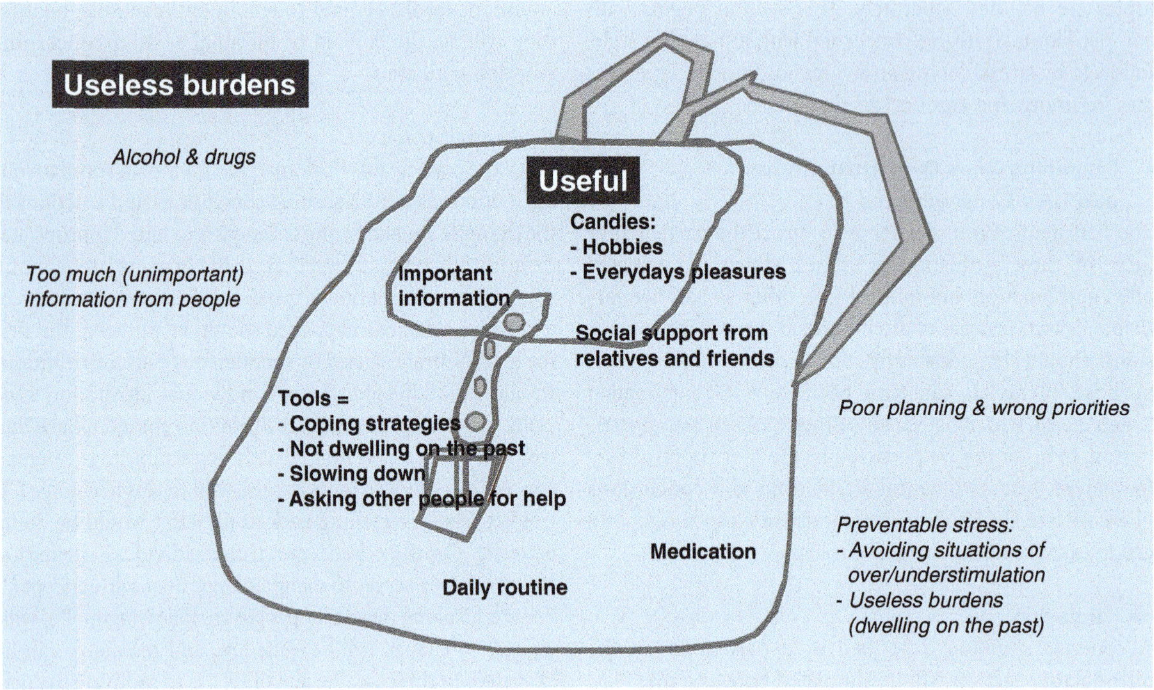

Fig. 2.28 "My personal rucksack" (vulnerability/stress model): example from an INT group

viewing and explaining events. On the basis of ▶ CD Information Sheet 39, participants finally fill out ▶ CD Worksheet 24 ("Examining my causal attribution") individually using an example situation from ▶ CD Materials 19–21. To activate the participants, the example situation, determined beforehand by the therapists, can also be performed as a role play. It is then recommended to motivate several group members to take over the active role. The participants should compare and contrast the spontaneously expressed attributions they made in the simulated situation. Inappropriate false attributions should be replaced with alternative attributions and applied in the role play. This intervention concludes with an extensive final discussion of the conclusions and consequences of different causal attributions in a situation. This promotes self-reflection and the active generation of alternative explanations and will be applied repeatedly in the following restitution section.

Strategies for Stress Reduction

As explained already in the introductory section, attributions are often interconnected with one's personal experience of stress. Now that participants have learned reattribution strategies, techniques for coping with stress can be discussed. Building on the vulnerability/stress model (see ▶ CD Information Sheet 37 "Vulnerability and stress"), first the relation between vulnerability and stress is reiterated. With a view to personal vulnerability and strains to be overcome, the patient's own experience of illness is designated as a life journey and compared with a mountain hike. This metaphor, also used in psychoeducational approaches (Roder et al. 2008b), is described on ▶ CD Information Sheet 40 ("Mountain hike"). This compares vulnerability with the physical constitution of a hiker, individual strains with the contents of the hiker's rucksack, and finally coping behavior with packing and carrying the rucksack. The greater the weight of the rucksack is, the greater the strain and stress. Preventative coping with strain consists of

- reducing strain (distinguishing useful and useless articles in the hiker's rucksack),
- asking for help (asking another hiker about the path), and
- applying effective coping strategies and thereby increasing the threshold of vulnerability (leaving useless burdens at home before hiking).

Figure 2.28 shows an example of a "rucksack model" developed in an INT group.

Stress-coping strategies are also developed for individual application. These are easy to learn and use and serve as supplements to emergency medication in case of severe stress. One central element of this intervention is the habituation of these strategies via repeated practice as indicated later in the restitution section. Yet the stress-coping strategies introduced in the following are not

	Stressor	Person	Reaction
	Change the stressor	**Change yourself**	**Reduce agitation**
Short-term strategies	• withdrawal	• *not possible!*	• **relaxation (breathing)** • **stopping our thoughts** • **self-verbalization** • **shaping attention**
Long-term strategies	• solving the problem • time management • avoid overly challenging situations	• cognitive restructuring • improving social competence • re-learning positive activities and enjoyment • acquiring protective life habits • activities that prevent stress (leisure time)	• regular relaxation exercises

Fig. 2.29 Strategies for coping with stress (Roder et al. 2008b, modified; with kind permission of Hans Huber Verlag)

meant primarily to prevent recurrence. Rather, they serve to enable the persons concerned to interrupt their own reactions to internally or externally induced stress. Only once mutually reinforcing reactions on cognitive, emotional, physical, and behavioral levels (a "vicious circle") are interrupted is one capable of applying suitable strategies for coping with a stressful or problematic situation. The recommended didactic procedure is first to sketch the model of the "vicious circle of anxiety" often used in behavior therapy and to accompany it with concrete examples.

Example

In stress-inducing situations, we often immediately react with a negative feeling (e.g., fear or rage), which is accompanied by spontaneous thought (e.g.,"I can't do that!","I'm lost!","I have to get out of here!"). These are accompanied by physical reactions (e.g., rapid heartbeat, tightness in the chest, trembling, intense sweating) and finally lead to consequences in behavior such as walking restlessly back and forth or becoming rigid. These different reactions can reinforce each other and maximize stress. For example: When we notice tightness in the chest, this increases our feeling of anxiety and our thoughts start racing.

The "vicious circle" being described here should be drawn on the flip chart. References to possible stress-coping strategies are made at different points interrupting the "vicious circle".

Example

It would be useful to interrupt this vicious circle so that feelings, thought, physical sensations, and behavioral reactions no longer reinforce each other. It would be good to be able to stop our thoughts, reduce negative feelings, and calm ourselves down. How is this possible?

At this point, therapists can ask for and compile participants' experiences in coping with concrete everyday situations involving stress. The literature cites a variety of possible coping strategies for stress reduction. Figure 2.29 summarizes a few selected examples that have proven effective and easily applicable for schizophrenia patients. These strategies have already been described in detail by our team elsewhere (Roder et al. 2008b). Figure 2.29 also helps the therapists to classify participants' experiences of coping with stress. In the following, the short-term coping strategies on the reaction side, which the participants can apply immediately, are of particular interest. These should now be presented in order to support self-help. For this purpose, ► CD Information Sheet 41 ("Coping with stress by yourself") is available on the accompanying ► CD-ROM. It summarizes the four strategies of breathing deeply, stopping thoughts, self-verbalization, and attention control. Group members first practice each strategy individually. Each finds at least three sentences (self-verbalization) that suit him or her. The four strategies are then practiced repeatedly and in combination (e.g., deep breathing – stopping thoughts – self-verbalization). In the restitution section, these stress-coping strategies will be further habituated and transferred to everyday life by means of independent exercises.

Strategies for Emotion Regulation

Using ► CD Information Sheet 38 as a basis, the primary therapist and the participants first develop a simple model of emotion regulation (Groß 1998). In this model, emotional reactions represent the consequence of situational triggers (situation). These triggers can be internal or external. Whether we react to a situation depends on which of these situational stimulants we direct our attention to, thereby perceiving them (attention processes). The next step is to interpret the situation (evaluation processes) and the associated emotional reaction. It is important that the therapist stresses the relation between this topic and the previously discussed areas of selective attention and attribution. The model should also be put in concrete terms using everyday examples provided by the patients. If they are unable to supply their own examples, ► CD Vignette 17 can also be utilized for this purpose.

The group then develops possible strategies of emotion regulation. These can be inserted at various points of the process model (Groß and Thompson 2007) (► CD Information Sheet 42):

Selecting the Situation

One possible strategy is to avoid situations, persons, or objects which we know to be triggers of certain emotions. To do this, it is necessary that we are able to anticipate the emotional consequences of a situation. This treatment unit should focus in particular on selecting situations that induce positive emotions. For example, it can be helpful to meet friends, plan a day trip, or go to a café when we are feeling sad or anxious in order to induce positive emotions. Situations that trigger anxiety or annoyance (large crowds of people, for example) can be avoided in order to reduce acute emotional strain as quickly as possible. This avoidance behavior can also help perpetuate the problem, however. Therefore, it should become clear to the participants that strategies that result in long-term positive emotions are preferable to those that only grant short-term relief by avoiding the situation. One example of this is purposely seeking an angst-ridden situation in order to experience that the feared consequences do not arise.

Changing the Situation

This strategy aims to alter an external situation in such a way that its emotional effect is also modified. For example, it can be easier to seek out an anxiety-inducing or aggravating situation if friends are there for support. Participants should thus plan carefully under what circumstances they can better master situations.

Changing Attention Processes

Controlling attention is a valuable strategy of emotion regulation. The focus of our attention decides what information we perceive and thus affects our emotional reactions. The technique of attention control proves especially helpful when the situation cannot be modified. Various techniques of attention control are suitable for this:

- Distraction by thought and actions (e.g., listening to music).
- Selective attention on positive aspects of the situation and on other sources of information (e.g., precise observation of particular details of the situation). This requires that the person can detach himself or herself from the emotional focus.

Changing Evaluation Processes

This strategy begins with the interpretation of a situation involving personal experiences and expectations. Various cognitive variation techniques are used (such as cognitive restructuring and positive reframing) to change the significance of an event or the assessment of our coping resources. The final aim is to alter our emotional reaction to the situation (e.g., questioning the nonverbal signals of others and not automatically assuming them to be devaluating).

Changing Emotional Reactions

While the above strategies concentrated on emotional triggers, now we focus on modifying emotional reactions. This can be approached on different levels:

- **Mental level:** remembering situations in which the person felt happy and safe and which the person coped with successfully; relaxing images; positive self-instructions ("I will not let myself be provoked by others. I will stay calm!"); re-evaluating the situation as non-threatening using new information or by changing the emphasis on existing information ("This situation is actually not nearly as threatening as I thought. I misinterpreted others' reactions as hostile.")
- **Physiological level:** relaxation exercises such as breathing exercises (inhaling and exhaling slowly and deeply) and muscle relaxation (tightening and relaxing particular muscles, stretching, making fists); upright posture
- **Behavioral level:** making contrary facial expressions (e.g., when angry); expressing emotions (e.g., when angry: shadow boxing, boxing with a sandbag, screaming, going to a gym; when sad: writing diary); suppressing expressive behavior by recognizing warning signals of undesired emotions (e.g., anger).

The therapist works on these strategies with the participants. The group then thinks about various emotional states they would like to change. These are noted on the flip chart, and together the group defines the desired target emotions. The group discusses which strategies are deployable. In a group exercise, emotion-triggering situations are reconstructed. The strategies are applied and assessed in terms of probability of success.

2.3.4.2.3 Restitution

The restitution section is organized into two parts: In the first part, spontaneous attributions are questioned with the help of various materials and alternatives are generated. In the second part, individualized stress-coping and emotion-regulation strategies are practiced further. In both sections, participants should fill out ▶ CD Worksheet 4 ("My helpful strategies for…") before repeating each exercise.

▪ Attributions

In the following, participants practice analyzing spontaneous causal attributions repeatedly. ▶ CD Information Sheets 35, 36, and 39 as well as ▶ CD Worksheet 24 serve as the basis for the repeated practice of coping strategies. The didactic procedure is split into four stages. Stages 1–3 encompass the processing of verbally described situations on the accompanying ▶ CD-ROM (▶ CD Materials 19–21). Participants must first spontaneously name and then question causes for the scene being described. Stage 4 involves analyzing video sequences. All four levels will be described in more detail in the following.

▪▪ Stage 1

Described situations without direct interaction with a given causal attribution: Each participant receives a printout of an example situation (▶ CD Materials 19a–g). Each situation describes a situation with Peter. The participants first make an oral or written summary of the situation in their own words. Peter's given hypothesis is first analyzed in the group from his perspective. Then the group looks for alternative hypotheses for explaining the event and describes possible functional consequences. Spontaneous and alternative hypotheses are compared by making a reality check (▶ CD Information Sheet 39). Participants should be encouraged throughout to make personal connections to their everyday lives ("Have you had experiences of this in your everyday life? How would you react if you were in Peter's shoes? In order to illustrate the aforementioned attribution processes and functional consequences, it is recommended to act out the example situations in role plays.

▪▪ Stage 2

Described situations with direct interaction with a given causal attribution: Each participant receives a printout of an example situation with the protagonist Peter (▶ CD Materials 20a–g). In these situations, Peter is in direct contact with the persons he holds responsible for the event being described. His spontaneous hypothesis is also given. The rest of the procedure is identical to that of stage 1.

▪▪ Stage 3

Described situations with direct interaction without a given causal attribution: As opposed to stage 2, these situations (▶ CD Materials 21a–k) do not provide a hypothesis. Instead, open questions on the cause of the event (hypotheses) and consequences are available. Because there is no predefined hypothesis, the connection to participants' personal daily lives is given greater emphasis. Participants' hypotheses can be communicated verbally or noted down on ▶ CD Materials 21. The participants compile and compare their hypotheses as in stages 1 and 2. Presenting the situation in the form of role plays is especially helpful for both understanding and self-reflection.

▪▪ Stage 4

Causal attribution in the role of the observer of a situation: Finally, causes of social interactions between other persons are to be defined and explained. The materials for this are the films described above. The objective is for the group to watch concise, often exaggeratedly played scenes in which common or surprising examples of interaction between characters are shown. The group then attempts to explain the action shown and to formulate possible consequences for the interaction partners involved (thoughts, feelings, physical and behavioral reactions). Again, the scenes can be reenacted later in role plays in case there are difficulties in understanding. Participants compare different explanatory hypotheses of an action. To check the validity of a hypothesis, it is possible to watch the following scenes of the film. This intervention is based on short film sequences, not on complete films. Module D factors in the cognitive functions that have already been worked on. The film scenes thus also serve as a final summary of the compensation strategies developed in Modules A–D. Here is a short overview of the films:

- "Analyze This"
- "Analyze That"
- "There's Something About Mary"
- "What about Bob?" ("What about Bob?")
- "Groundhog Day"
- "A Beautiful Mind"
- "Elling"
- "Mors Elling"
- "As Good as it Gets"

Of course, other films can be used as well.

▪ **Coping with Stress and Emotion Regulation**

In the restitution section, participants have many opportunities to practice individualized strategies of coping with stress and regulating emotion (▶ CD Information Sheets 40–42).

Stress-Coping Strategies The following exercise is one way to actively practice the strategy of deep breathing/stopping thoughts/self-verbalization on ▶ CD Information Sheet 41. The participants and therapists walk through the therapy room and recite their individual stress-coping techniques out loud. Physical contact is prohibited. By increasing the pace, the amount of stress can be intensified. The object of the exercise is to concentrate on one's stress-coping strategies in spite of sensory overload. If a participant is unsuccessful in this, she can withdraw to a quiet corner to apply her strategies there and recite them again.

Situations from Everyday Life One participant selects an everyday situation that triggers negative emotions. The person concerned describes the situation exactly and has two group members reenact it. Together, the group considers which strategies for improving emotion regulation could be helpful and why other strategies failed. The participant concerned can then assume his own role in the role play and rehearse the strategies.

2.3.4.2.4 In Vivo Exercises and Independent Exercises

The following is an example of an in vivo exercise that would help participants integrate strategies learned in the areas of attribution, stress-coping, and emotion regulation into their everyday lives. This exercise is a not very straining experience since the participants only assume the role of observers. Before starting the exercise, every group member fills out ▶ CD Worksheet 4 ("My helpful strategies for…"). The group goes to a crowded spot in the city with seating options and the possibility of retreat. Altogether or in smaller groups, the participants try to observe and explain the social interactions of passers-by. The focus should be on causal attributions and resulting conclusions. They can take notes in the process. After 20 or 30 min, the group confers for the first time about their observations and the attributions they drew from them. The participants should also report about their own experiences of stress, the emotional strain involved in the observer role, and the application of coping strategies (▶ CD Worksheet 4). The next group session starts with an extensive discussion of the exercise.

In addition, the participants are also motivated to do individual exercises and homework. For this purpose, they themselves can select everyday examples from the areas of "walking around town", "shopping day", "meeting friends and family", and "work relationships". It is important that the participants choose single, clearly defined situations and that they plan and prepare it with the help of the worksheets (▶ CD Worksheet 5). Individualized strategies for coping with stress and emotion should be practiced repeatedly. The independent exercises are especially suitable for this purpose. The group can then have a detailed discussion of the stress and straining emotions resulting from the attributions made during the independent exercises. It is also a good opportunity to involve previously learned strategies for other neurocognitive and social-cognitive functions in the independent exercises. This final integration of all the compensation strategies requires especially thorough preparation and debriefing.

2.4 Example Organization of 30 INT Sessions

In the following, a record was made of an INT group consisting of 30 sessions of 90 min each in order to illustrate the didactic method, content, progress of the treatment. The scope of the 30 sessions largely corresponded to the diagnostic evaluation of the 5–8 participants. This was a homogeneous group consisting of participants with group experience, some with excellent resources with deficits in cognitive functioning in only a few areas. If group members are more diverse and suffer from more intense functional deficits, one can assume that the treatment duration will be longer and that the therapy content will have to be altered to some extent.

Each session is described briefly and assigned to one of the four therapy areas (Modules A–D). Each topic area merges seamlessly with the next. The content of the next topic already begins while processing of the previous topic is still being concluded. Exercises for independent execution and in vivo exercises are only mentioned occasionally as examples.

▪ **Module A: Speed of Information Processing and Attention – Emotional Perception (7 Sessions)**

▪▪ **Session 1: Introduction to the Group and to the Area of Speed of Information Processing**

- Short overview of therapy contents, getting to know each other and establishing group rules.
- Introduction to the area of speed of information processing.
- Promote self-perception using the first CogPack exercises (e.g., VISUMOTOR). Conversation about knowledge/previous experience with computers

(No pressure! Anyone can do it!) Pep talk on giving mutual support by means of positive feedback.
After every exercise, the results are observed and improvements and reinforced.
- Feedback session: Was the exercise stimulating? Did I like it? Did I find myself fast/slow?
- Assessment of own cognitive profile in the target area (worksheet).
- Quick feedback round.

This can be done at the end of each session, but it is not mandatory, so it will not be referred to in the following exercises.

Session 2: Introduction to the Areas of Speed and Attention/Vigilance

- Short check-in. Refresh the first session: The contents of the last lesson are summarized as a memory exercise.
  This exercise will be performed at the beginning of every session from now on (and will not be mentioned anymore in the following sessions).
- The influence of alertness: Establish connection to participants' everyday lives by reading the associated vignettes as a group. Segue to the CogPack exercise: Did I feel alert or tired during the exercise? How would my speed change if I felt more alert?
- Introduce the topics of attention and vigilance and read associated vignettes.

Session 3: Introduction to Factors Influencing Speed of Information Processing and Attention/Vigilance

- The influence of interest: exercise with current newspapers or magazines. Participants select one of several newspapers or magazines. They can then flip through them and should observe where their own attention lingers. Discussion of texts and pictures, which met with the interest of individual participants. Activation of resources.
- The influence of daily rhythm: worksheet: "Alertness and speed/attention": presentation of a typical daily chart of the degree of temporary alertness. Participants then fill out their own charts individually. Determine individual times of day and situations in which fatigue is a problem. Sensitize participants for desires and possibilities of change.
- Introduce influential factors of medication, motivation, and mood and process them using materials

Session 4: Compensation and Restitution in the Areas of Speed of Information Processing and Attention/Vigilance

- Developing different behavioral-therapeutic techniques (e.g., active breaks, self-verbalizations) as compensation strategies
- First experiences of the participants in applying coping strategies in group exercises (therapy materials: IPT card-sorting exercise and the "speed" card-sorting exercise).
- Make a connection to everyday life via the specific spheres of living, work, and recreation under consideration of patients' individual sleep/wake rhythm.
- Move to computer room; short computer practice (15 min) of compensation strategies (CogPack, e.g., the exercises PIECE-WORK, UFO, FALLING STARS).
- Give the group an independent exercise (e.g., self-observation in the target area).

Session 5: Restitution in the Areas of Speed and Attention/Vigilance – Introduction to Emotional Perception

- Feedback on independent exercise: problem analysis and reinforcement of success experiences.
- Repeated computer practice of compensation strategies for the neurocognitive target areas (max. 30 min); subsequent discussion of the exercises: How did I experience this exercise? Was it exciting or boring? How fast was I? How long was I able to concentrate? What coping strategies were helpful to me?
- Check the initial self-assessment of performance in the target areas.
- Move to the group room: introduction to emotional perception with information sheets (filter model, definition of basic emotions) and a vignette (reference to personal, everyday life).
- Self-assessment of performance in the target area of emotional perception (worksheet).

Session 6: Restitution in the Target Areas of Speed, Attention/Vigilance and Compensation in the Area of Emotional Perception

- Collect strategies for affect decoding (facial expressions, gestures, posture) in group discussion and supplement using information sheets.
- Affect decoding in three stages: use the Ekman picture series and available e-materials. Important in group discussion: distinguishing between facts and spontaneous assumptions/assertions.

- Restitution of the neurocognitive section: The last 15–30 min are dedicated to repeating the CogPack exercises and/or card-sorting exercises (IPT, speed). Final review of initial assessment of own performance in the target area.

Session 7: Restitution in the Area of Emotional Perception

- Card-sorting exercise on emotional concept formation
- Restitution: re-distribution of e-materials on affect decoding.
- Check self-assessment of performance in the target area.
- Independent exercise (e.g., observing and noting everyday emotional expression of familiar persons).

Module B: Verbal and Visual Learning and Memory – Social Perception (6 Sessions)

Session 8: Introduction and Compensation in the Areas of Learning and Memory

- Feedback on previous independent exercise (emotional perception).
- Introduction to verbal and visual memory using information sheets (types and contents of memory, storage model) and vignette (reference to personal, everyday life).
- Beginning of the compensation section: collection of compensation strategies previously implemented by participants.

Session 9: Compensation and Restitution in the Areas of Learning and Memory

- Short check-in; refresh the last session.
- Develop further compensation strategies for improving memory using information sheets (verbal memory, memorizing textual and conversational contents, number memory, visual memory, prospective memory) and initial application in corresponding group exercises.
- Move to the group room: Practice compensation strategies developed in the group with CogPack exercises for the different memory contents (e.g., MEMORY).

Session 10: Restitution in the Areas of Learning and Memory

- Further CogPack exercises (e.g., NEW-or-NOT, ARCHIVE, ON-THE-ROAD, EYEWITNESS, READING). Participants consciously apply compensation strategies to test which strategies suit them better. The computer exercises should be discussed extensively afterwards.
- In the second part of the session, group exercises are performed using available materials (e.g., memorizing lists of words, names, and numbers; interactive exercise "new identity"; memorizing textual information).
- Finally, participants are instructed to perform an independent memory exercise at home (e.g., memorizing the names of neighbors).

Session 11: Restitution in the Areas of Learning and Memory – Introduction to the Areas of Social Perception and Perspective Adoption

- Feedback on independent memory exercise.
- Restitution for the areas of learning and memory (session 10, 2nd part)
- Introduction and definition of social perception and perspective adoption (ToM) using information sheets (situation-appropriate recognition of information, distinguishing between facts and assumptions, empathy) and a vignette (connection to everyday life).
- Self-assessment of performance in the target area (worksheet).

Session 12: Compensation in the Areas of Social Perception and Perspective Adoption

- Strategies for improving social perception in three steps using visual stimuli (IPT pictures): collecting information, interpretation, finding a title
- Refer the depicted situations to participants' everyday lives. The situations can be acted out in role plays (Have I also experienced such situations? What happened in my case? How did I behave?).
- Try to adopt the perspective of the persons being depicted (How does that person feel? What does he/she think? Which facts give evidence for me assumption?),
- If participants have difficulties with the emotional expressions contained on the IPT pictures, the affect decoding strategies should be reviewed briefly using associated visual materials from Module A.

Session 13: Compensation and Restitution in the Areas of Social Perception and Perspective Adoption

- Group exercise on social perspective adoption using therapy materials (materials with example situations, e-materials on perspective adoptions with the three topics of "cities", "water", and "people". One half of

the group describes a target picture; the other has to identify the described picture from 30 topically similar ones).
- Analysis of film excerpts (What is this about? What is the basic message of the film clip?).
- Repeated processing of other IPT pictures.
- Check the initial self-assessment of functioning in the target area (worksheet).

Module C: Reasoning and Problem Solving – Social Schemas (8 Sessions)

Session 14: Introduction to the Areas of Reasoning and Problem Solving
- Introduction and definition of the areas of reasoning (cognitive flexibility and concept formation) and problem solving (target/problem orientation: target/actual state) using information sheets and a vignette (connection to participants' everyday life).
- Make reference to speed of information processing, attention, and memory (Modules A and B) as prerequisites for well-functioning reasoning and problem-solving capabilities.
- Group exercises for demonstration and to collect experiences in dealing with the target cognitive functions.
- Self-assessment of performance in the target area.

Session 15: Introduction and Compensation in the Areas of Reasoning and Problem Solving
- Identification of factors influencing reasoning and problem solving (information sheet).
- Barriers to realizing goals in participants' everyday lives.
- Develop coping strategies for improving goal-realization: problem-solving model in 6 steps (information sheet).
- Further group exercise on the target area (materials).
- Individual exercise on goal-realization with respect to everyday personal problems which appear to be realistically solvable. Each participant identifies at least one individual problem (defining the target), which is discussed turn by turn within the group. Implementation of the solution strategies developed in the group takes place between the sessions and requires extensive preliminary and concluding discussion. This intervention extends over the following sessions.

Session 16: Compensation in the Area of Problem Solving
- Debrief independently implemented strategies for goal-realization (problem analysis, determining alternative solution strategies).
- Talk about individualized problems as yet to be discussed in the group and develop solution strategies.

Session 17: Compensation and Restitution in the Area of Problem Solving
- Debrief independently implemented strategies for goal-realization (problem analysis, determining alternative solution strategies).
- Develop strategies for goal-oriented action planning (information sheet) and application in group exercises (materials).
- Move to the group room: application of developed compensation strategies in CogPack exercises (e.g., SCALES, LABYRINTHS).

Session 18: Compensation in the Area of Reasoning – Restitution in the Areas of Reasoning and Problem Solving
- Debrief independently implemented strategies for goal-realization (problem analysis, determining alternative solution strategies).
- Develop compensation strategies with respect to "How can I better find the right words?" (concept formation).
- Group exercises provide initial experiences in implementing developed strategies (materials).
- Move to the group room: repeated application of developed compensation strategies in CogPack exercises (e.g., SCALES, LABYRINTHS, ANAGRAMS, GUESSWORDS, CONCEPTS).

Session 19: Restitution in the Areas of Reasoning and Problem Solving – Introduction to the Area of Social Schemas
- Debrief independently implemented strategies for goal-realization (problem analysis, determining alternative solution strategies).
- Repeated practice of individualized strategies for problem solving, action planning, and concept formation – alternately in group exercises and computer exercises (CogPack exercises partially in teams of two or as a competition between two halves of the group).
- Check initial self-assessments in the target areas (worksheet).
- Introduction and definition of social schemas (social rules and roles) using information sheets and a vignette (connection to everyday lives).
- Make direct connection between social schemas and reasoning, problem solving, and action planning. Social schemas contain action sequences and prejudices in social contexts.

- Self-assessment of performance in the target area (worksheet).
- Topics of prejudice and stigmatization: participant experiences.

Session 20: Compensation in the Area of Social Schemas

- Debrief independently implemented strategies for goal-realization (problem analysis, determining alternative solution strategies).
- Identify social rules and roles (information sheet "How do I recognize that my behavior doesn't conform to rules?").
- Strategies for coping with stigmatization and being able to distance oneself (information sheets and worksheets) are tried out in role plays.

Session 21: Compensation and Restitution in the Area of Social Schemas

- Group exercises on social action sequences and action planning (social scripts: therapy materials).
- Analyze social schemas in film excerpts (violation of and adherence to social rules).
- Check the initial self-assessment of functioning in the target area (worksheet).

Module D: Working Memory and Attribution/Emotion Regulation (9 Sessions)

Session 22: Introduction to the Area of Working Memory

- Introduction to and definition of working memory using worksheet (working memory as control center, functioning during sensory overload, selective attention) and a vignette (connection to everyday life).
- Refer back to previous functional areas as prerequisites for direct processing in working memory (e.g., attention, verbal and visual memory).
- Self-assessment of performance in the target area (worksheet).

Session 23: Compensation in the Area of Working Memory

- Develop strategies for coping with distraction and hyperactivation caused by sensory overload (information sheets and worksheets).
- Assess one's own automatic action rituals for coping with internal and external sensory overload (cost/benefit calculation, decision aids).
- First application of new strategies for preventing distraction and hyperactivation in group exercises (materials).
- Alternating between several actions Strategies for letting go of one action and moving on to another (worksheet and materials).

Session 24: Compensation and Restitution in the Area of Working Memory

- Selective attention. Strategies for reducing distraction, also during conversation (information sheets and materials). Practice strategies in role plays.
- Transition to the restitution section: various group exercises (e.g., matchstick exercise (learning strategies), card-sorting exercise (cognitive flexibility), carrying out several activities at once (Action change; materials), picture series on selective perception (materials) alternate in blocks with computer exercises (CogPack: e.g., SEARCH, CONNECT, MONEY, INTERFERENCE, COLORS&LABELS).

Session 25: Restitution in the Area of Working Memory

- Continuation of the restitution section from session 24: group exercises and computer exercises in blocks of 20–30 min with debriefing
- Check previous self-assessment of performance in the target area.
- Final preliminary discussion of an already announced group in vivo exercise outside the therapy room during the next (time-wise slightly longer) session. The group decides in this context to make an excursion together to a nearby department store. The following was defined as an individual goal: each participant should make a list in advance of things concerning which he/she will ask for information on location (e.g., curtains for the kitchen, clothing, mobile phone, etc.). Another objective is to ask for directions to the appropriate department despite sensory overload and to speak to the relevant salesperson in order to obtain the information needed.

This in vivo exercise may push some participants' limits of strain resistance. For this reason, it is indispensable that participants are adequately prepared (e.g., by role play) and each have written notes and that therapists offer assistance.

Session 26: In Vivo Exercise in the Area of Working Memory

- Short preparation of the forthcoming exercise discussed already in the last session.
- Field trip to the department store. The group splits up, each half being accompanied by one of the

therapists. A quiet meeting place is decided upon (e.g., the exit area or cafeteria of the department store as a withdrawal possibility). If a participant is having difficulties, the therapist assists and distracts him/her from the stress-inducing situation by means of conversation.
- After the exercise, there is a detailed debriefing session (Did I reach my goal? How was I able to cope with sensory overload and distraction? What did I think and feel? Did I experience a lot of stress?). The debriefing session can also take place at the beginning of the next session if circumstances require.

▪▪ Session 27: Introduction and Compensation in the Area of Attribution
- Introduction to and definition of attributions using a worksheet (spontaneous and external causal attribution and conclusion processes) and a vignette (connection to everyday life).
- Self-assessment of performance in the target area (worksheet).
- Group discussion on potential factors influencing the individual attribution process (information sheet).
- Place the focus on one's own attribution style and question one's own spontaneous attributions and their consequences (worksheet, information sheets).
- Reattribution: replace spontaneous attributions with alternative causal attributions and compare the consequences (group exercise).

▪▪ Session 28: Restitution in the Area of Attribution
- Reattribution in 4 stages: situations without interaction with given causal attribution, situations with interaction with given causal attribution, situations with interaction without given causal attribution, causal attribution from the role of observer.
- Repetition of group exercise on social attributions using materials on the accompanying ▶ CD-ROM and film clips.
- Check the initial self-assessment of functioning in the target area (worksheet).

▪▪ Session 29: Introduction and Compensation in the Area of Emotion Regulation
- Introduction to and definition of "emotion regulation" using a worksheet (vulnerability/stress model, model of emotion regulation) and a vignette (connection to everyday life).
- Self-assessment of performance in the target area (worksheet).
- Refer back to previous areas of neurocognitive and social-cognitive functioning, in which emotional strains and experiences of stress were mentioned as individual treatment goals but were initially put aside.
- Self-assessment of own ability to cope with stress and straining emotions (worksheet).
- Development and initial practice of stress-coping and emotion-regulation strategies (information sheets).
- Independent exercise between sessions: application of learned coping strategies in real situation of participants' individual everyday life.

▪▪ Session 30: Restitution in the Area of Emotion Regulation – Conclusion of Treatment
- Debrief independent exercise (What problems did I have? How could I change my strategy?).
- Further practice of stress-coping and emotion-regulation strategies in group exercises.
- Conclusion of treatment: short recap of therapy contents. Where was I able to gain experience in coping? Did my self-assessments of cognitive performance in the various target areas of the four modules change? (worksheet).
- Feedback session on the therapy with the therapy team and the participants.
- Now what? Networking and indication of further treatment options during "coffee and cake".

2.5 Motivation Building, Forming Relationships, and Group Processes

2.5.1 Building Motivation and Forming Relationships

Persons diagnosed with schizophrenia appear as a rule to be only conditionally, slightly, or not at all motivated for treatment options. For this reason, therapeutic interaction – one-on-one and in a group – requires special competencies. This is true both for the therapist performing the treatment and the referring personal physician. These competencies will be described briefly in the following. In these explanations, it is assumed that the primary therapist of the INT group is also the responsible personal therapist. If this is not the case, close cooperation is required between the referring physician and the primary therapist responsible for the group.

Before a patient takes part in an INT group, the therapist invites him to preliminary talks in a one-on-one setting. These talks comprise about 1–5 appointments of 30–45 min over a maximum of 4 weeks. The number of appointments depends on the level of motivation of the participant concerned. If there is little to no motivation and/or insight in the current problem and life situation, the therapist needs more time to build up motivation. 30–45 min appears to be an optimal length for the talks so as not to overtax the patient's information intake and to avoid excessively rapid and pronounced emotional stimulation. The beginning of the conversation is mainly positive and resource-oriented (e.g., making honest compliments, talking about positive experiences). Possible ways to improve behavior and experience can be addressed in a gradual way later. Discussion of deficits should be avoided.

The talks encompass the following objectives:

- giving hope, reinforcing intrinsic motivation to change
- discussing and clarifying resources
- accepting and encouraging
- building up positive, valuing interaction
- explaining, informing, making common decisions
- promoting self-efficacy and independence

▪ Giving Hope, Reinforcing Intrinsic Motivation to Change

The willingness to change can be inspired more easily if a person finds new hope that an apparently hopeless situation can take a turn for the better. For this reason, the therapist communicates positive possibilities for change in small, realistic steps – thus giving new ground for hope. Each patent shows intrinsic motivation for (changing) some personal area or other. This motivation, specific to each person, should be identified and reinforced (e.g., be with other people more; learn one's own vocation; live independently). Intrinsic motivation can be further encouraged in conversation with the therapist and embedded into INT's therapeutic interventions. Then patients have thoughts such as "If I complete INT, it will help me have more successful contact with others."

▪ Discussing and Clarifying Resources

Every person is in possession of resources, independent of how serious the mental disorder or illness might be. They only have to be activated and become perceivable to the person concerned. This is the task of the therapist. Resources might include: taking walks, playing certain games, helping others, doing small tasks, wanting to learn something. In our experience, resources should be activated to help form positive relationships at the beginning of the treatment. This also reinforces and consolidates therapeutic contact during tense, disharmonious moments of treatment. Therapeutic relationship formation is more of a complementary process here.

▪ Accepting and Encouraging/Building up Positive, Valuing Interaction

In the preliminary talks as well as later during group therapy, patients should have the feeling that the therapist accepts them unconditionally as a subject and thus as a unique person. Creating an atmosphere of positive and valuing communication and interaction is especially crucial to reach this objective (see e.g., "Motivational Discussions" by Miller and Rollnick 2009). Such an atmosphere provides the basis for a sustainable (group) therapy relationship, within which a patient can carefully venture his or her initial steps towards change. In group therapy, this basic approach also requires a considerable amount of group cohesion. Therefore, this basic therapeutic approach is not so much a therapeutic technique as, in our opinion, a basic ethical approach for therapists when interacting with patients.

▪ Explaining, Informing, Making Common Decisions

Furthermore, open and information-based therapeutic discussion also contributes to a sound and sustainable therapeutic relationship. In the preliminary talks and during group therapy, patients are carefully and precisely informed about the therapeutic goals and steps and involved in associated, goal-oriented decisions. It is important that the therapist recognizes how much clear and explicit information, transparency, and room for decision-making can be expected of a particular patient. It is practical to distinguish between short-term, medium-term, and long-term (therapeutic) goals (see ▶ Chap. 4). In any case, short-term goals should be communicated well and clearly and find mutual acceptance.

▪ Promoting Self-Efficacy and Independence

During preliminary talks, the therapist stresses that participation in an INT group should lead to more self-efficacy (e.g., realizing one's own wants and goals) and independence (e.g., having to contact fewer health care persons).

If – perhaps after participating in a trial session – the person concerned has decided to join the group, his or her level of motivation must be further maintained. The basic therapeutic approach and structured group guidance help achieve this (▶ Sect. 2.5.2), as does INT's didactic structure itself. The highly varied therapeutic interventions (using various therapy materials), the gradual adjustment of therapy content to patients' individual level of strain and performance (reduction of errors), participants' freedom of choice in many of the individualized interventions, and the topics' strict relevance to everyday life have all proved to be advantageous factors in promoting and maintaining motivation.

It should be stressed again at this point that implementing the INT program requires more than specific therapeutic techniques. The therapist's basic ethical attitude, as described above, is also a key factor. This basic therapeutic approach helps to build up a good level of

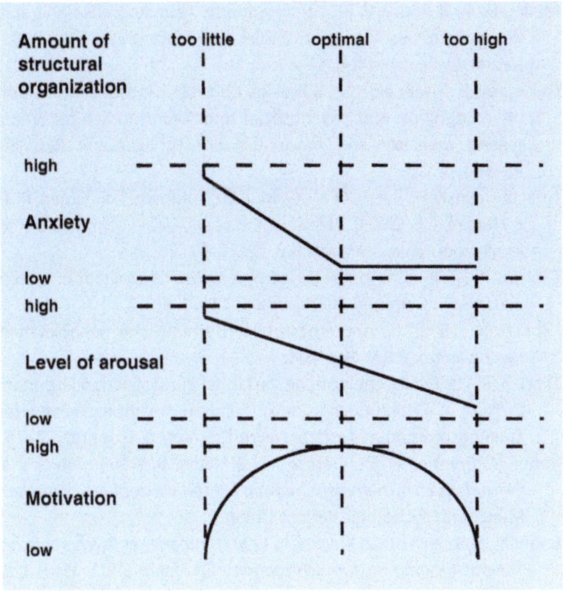

Fig. 2.30 Anxiety, activation, and motivation as structuring functions in groups of patients with schizophrenia (Roder et al. 2008a; with kind permission of Beltz Verlag)

motivation and a therapeutic relationship that is sustainable for the middle or long term. We thus advise expressly against interpreting INT exclusively as an application of therapeutic techniques in the sense of a "training course" lasting only a few sessions.

2.5.2 Group Processes

Conducting groups made up of persons with schizophrenia places special demands on group therapists. It is particularly important that well-structured exercises are used as well as an equally well-structured therapeutic style for building up a favorable group atmosphere. This solidifies group cohesion. This is especially true at the start of the group, when the participants are not yet acquainted with each other. Structuring, anxiety, motivation, and psychophysiological activation (independent variables) need to be seen in close connection with the respective structure (independent variable) that is predominant in the group. On the basis of our clinical experience, the following conclusions can be made for groups of persons affected by schizophrenia (Fig. 2.30).

A group works optimally (focused concentration on tasks and topic; the highest possible motivation) when anxiety levels are very low (or there is no anxiety at all) and the activation level is average. The spectrum of topics is also of interest to participants. The structure is adjusted to the requirements of the group (optimal structuring). If group anxiety levels are high however (excessive challenge), the result is usually a high level of activation not focused on the task. Participant resistance to participating in the group (motivation) can be pronounced. There is no structure, or it is too limited. If, on the contrary, a group is excessively structured, the level of anxiety may indeed be quite low (or there may be no anxiety at all). However, resistance to cooperation may result again since there is no more motivation (insufficient challenge). The group's activation level is then almost zero. So the therapist has to try to regulate these four areas (motivation, anxiety, activation level, structure) by careful observation and perception of the group process. The following procedures are possible options for strengthening group structure:

- leader-centered communication style
- directive discussion
- addressing group members by name
- not allowing longer period of silence to occur
- task-centered, topic-centered method
- establishing group rules and norms
- giving feedback for all participant contributions
- summarizing
- objectively oriented group contents
- no interpretations of ambiguities
- predicting the group process

Every group session can be divided into three phases:

1. Warm-up phase
2. Topic-centered phase
3. Final phase

During the first, somewhat short phase (5–10 min), the therapist creates a relaxed, anxiety-free, and sustainable group atmosphere. This makes it possible for the participants to work in a task-centered, topic-centered way. In doing this, the therapist can provide a quick overview of the topics of the session and (positively) address each participant briefly, e.g., to ask how he or she is doing ("joining"). In the topic-centered phase, the therapists introduce the topics selected for the session and develop them. During the (short) final phase, a positive group feeling is established; the therapist clears up any uncertainties, strains, or stresses. This can be achieved by making a summarizing review while highlighting positive aspects of the session. At the same time, the therapist can motivate the participants by previewing the next group session. The techniques of "reframing" and "positive connotation" have proven useful and helpful again and again for establishing a positive group atmosphere. In reframing, the therapist puts a certain event into a new, more positive context. Positive connotation involves emphasizing the positive aspects of a certain "problem". If (personal) problems are discussed, (positive), empathetic feedback (sympathy; "sharing") by other group members can help the person with the problem feel better understood by the group. This usually leads to enhanced group cohesion.

References

Baddeley, A. D. (1986). *So denkt der Mensch*. München: Droemer-Knaur.

Barch, D., & Carter, C. (2005). Amphetamine improves cognitive function in medicated individuals with schizophrenia and in healthy volunteers. *Schizophr Res, 77*(1), 43–58.

Bäuml, J., & Pitschel-Walz, G. (2008). *Psychoedukation bei schizophrenen Erkrankungen* (2nd ed.). Stuttgart: Schattauer.

Bäuml J, Pitschel-Walz G, Berger H, Gunia H, Heinz A, Juckel G (2010) (2008) Arbeitsbuch PsychoEdukation bei Schizophrenie, 2. Auflage. Schattauer, Stuttgart

Ekman, P. (1993). Facial Expression and Emotion. *American Psychologist, 48*(4), 384–392.

Ekman, P., & Friesen, W. V. (1976). *Pictures of facial affect*. Palo Alto: Consulting Psychologists Press.

Green, M. F., & Nuechterlein, K. H. (2004). The MATRICS initiative: developing a consensus cognitive battery for clinical trials. *Schizophr Res, 72*, 1–3.

Green, M. F., Olivier, B., Crawley, J. N., Penn, D. L., & Silverstein, S. (2005). Social cognition in schizophrenia: recommendations from the measurement and treatment research to improve cognition in schizophrenia new approaches conference. *Schizophr Res, 31*, 882–887.

Groß, J. J. (1998). The emerging field of emotion regulation: an integrative review. *Rev Gen Psychol, 2*, 271–299.

Groß, J. J., & Thompson, R. A. (2007). Emotion regulation: conceptual foundations. In J. J. Groß (Ed.), *Handbook of emotion regulation* (pp. 3–24). New York: Guilford Press.

Hodel B (1998) Einschätzung von "Emotionsfotos": Auswertung der Daten. Unveröffentlichtes Arbeitspapier. Universitätslinik und Poliklinik für Psychiatrie, Bern

Kern, R. S., Liberman, R. P., Kopelowicz, A., Mintz, J., & Green, M. F. (2002). Applications of errorless learning for improving work performance in persons with schizophrenia. *Am J Psychiatry, 159*(11), 1921–1926.

Kern, R. S., Green, M. F., Mintz, J., & Liberman, R. P. (2003). Does 'errorless learning' compensate for neurocognitive impairments in the work rehabilitation of persons with schizophrenia? *Psychol Med, 33*(3), 433–442.

Kern, R. S., Green, M. F., Mitchell, S., Kopelowicz, A., Mintz, J., & Liberman, R. P. (2005). Extensions of errorless learning for social problem-solving deficits in schizophrenia. *Am J Psychiatry, 162*, 513–519.

MATRICS Assessment, Inc (2006) Matrics consensus cognitive battery (MCCB). Retrieved from http://www.matricsinc.org/MCCB.htm#1. Accessed May 2009

Medalia, A., & Thysen, J. (2008). Insight into neurocognitive dysfunction in schizophrenia. *Schizophr Bull, 24*, 1221–1230.

Miller, W. R., & Rollnick, S. (2009). *Motivierende Gesprächsführung* (3rd ed.). Freiburg: Lambertus.

Müller, D. R., & Roder, V. (2008). Empirical evidence for group therapy addressing social perception in schizophrenia. In J. B. Teiford (Ed.), *Social perception: 21st century issues and challenges* (pp. 51–80). New York: Nova.

Müller, D. R., & Roder, V. (2010). Integrated psychological therapy (IPT) and integrated neurocognitive therapy (INT). In V. Roder & A. Medalia (Eds.), *Neurocognition and social cognition in schizophrenia patients. Basic concepts and treatment* (pp. 118–144). Basel: Karger.

Müller, D. R., & Roder, V. (2012). Integrierte Neurokognitive Therapie. Kognitionen als Interventionsziel bei schizophren Erkrankten. *Neurol Psychiatrie, 14*(4), 57–63.

Nakagami, E., Xie, B., Hoe, M., & Brekke, J. S. (2008). Intrinsic motivation, neurocognition and psychosocial functioning in schizophrenia: testing mediator and moderator effects. *Schizophr Res, 105*, 95–104.

Nuechterlein, K. H., Barch, D. M., Gold, J. M., Goldberg, T. E., Green, M. F., & Heaton, T. E. (2004). Identification of separable cognitive factors in schizophrenia. *Schizophr Res, 72*, 29–39.

Olbrich, R. (1996). Computer based psychiatric rehabilitation: current activities in Germany. *Eur Psychiatry, 11*, 60–65.

Olbrich, R. (1998). Computergestutzte psychiatrische Rehabilitation. *Psychiatr Prax, 25*(3), 103–104.

Olbrich, R. (1999). Psychologische Verfahren zur Reduktion kognitiver Defizite. Erfahrungen mit einem computergestutzten Trainingsprogramm. *Fortschr Neurol Psychiatr, 67*(Suppl 2), 74–76.

Roder, V., Brenner, H. D., Kienzle, N., & Hodel, B. (1988). *Integriertes Psychologisches Therapieprogramm (IPT) für schizophrene Patienten*. München: Psychologie Verlags Union.

Roder, V., Brenner, H. D., & Kienzle, N. (2002). *Integriertes Psychologisches Therapieprogramm für schizophren Erkrankte (IPT)* (5th ed.). Weinheim: Beltz.

Roder, V., Brenner, H. D., & Kienzle, N. (2008a). *Integriertes Psychologisches Therapieprogramm bei schizophren Erkrankten IPT, 6. überarbeitete Auflage*. Weinheim: Beltz.

Roder, V., Zorn, P., Pfammatter, M., Andres, K., Brenner, H. D., & Müller, D. R. (2008b). *Praxishandbuch zur Verhaltenstherapeutischen Behandlung schizophren Erkrankter* (2nd ed.). Bern: Huber.

Roder, V., Müller, D. R., Brenner, H. D., & Spaulding, W. D. (2010). *Integrated Psychological Therapy (IPT) for the treatment of neurocognition, social cognition, and social competencies in schizophrenia patients*. Göttingen: Hogrefe.

Roder, V., Müller, D. R., & Schmidt, S. J. (2011). Effectiveness of the Integrated Psychological Therapy (IPT) for schizophrenia patients: a research up-date. *Schizophr Bull, 37*(Suppl 2), 71–79.

Schank, R. C., & Abelson, R. (1977). *Scripts, plans, goals, and understanding*. Hillsdale: Earlbaum Assoc.

Velligan, D. I., Kern, R. S., & Gold, J. M. (2006). Cognitive rehabilitation for schizophrenia and the putative role of motivation and expectancies. *Schizophr Bull, 32*, 474–485.

Therapy Requirements, Possible Applications, and Indication

D. R. Müller, V. Roder

Additional material (CD-ROM) to this book can be downloaded from http://extras.springer.com

V. Roder, D.R. Müller (eds.), *INT-Integrated Neurocognitive Therapy for Schizophrenia Patients*,
DOI 10.1007/978-3-319-13245-7_3,

The implementation of INT depends on various institutional conditions, which will be discussed in this chapter. In addition, the qualifications of the therapist team, characteristics and group composition of the patients have to be taken into account when planning an INT group. The chapter will conclude with a discussion from the point of view of differential indication of whether patients, on the basis of symptoms and treatment types, should be referred to INT or to other group interventions developed by our team. These include Integrated Psychological Therapy (IPT; Roder et al. 2008a, 2010) or the therapy programs targeting vocational, residential, and recreational domains (WAF; Roder et al. 2008b).

3.1 Setting Conditions

The general infrastructural requirements for implementing an INT group (room conditions, computers, materials) have already been addressed in ► Sect. 2.1. The question now is which types of institutions are suitable for INT's clinical implementation.

3.1.1 Types of Institutions

Hitherto, INT was implemented primarily in the context of outpatient and day-care treatment: outpatient clinics, day clinics, and (vocational) rehabilitation centers. Additionally, INT is also suitable as part of long-term treatment planning for the aftercare-treatment of patients currently treated in hospital. Such patients can already join the INT group before exiting the hospital and then continue to participate in the group after discharge. However, the requirements of group composition should be taken into account (► Sect. 3.3). Additional considerations need to be made with respect to local and institutional treatment options as well as the implementation type of open or closed groups.

3.1.2 Intra-institutional and Inter-institutional Options

Within the boundaries of local psychiatric care, it is sometimes difficult to recruit enough patients so that the optimal group size of five to eight participants is reached within a limited time frame. The therapists must then resort to recruiting patients from other institutes – for example, patients from different outpatient clinics and day clinics. Also, registered doctors and rehabilitation centers within a region often lack the opportunity to offer comparable (group) interventions. Assuming there is close collaboration between institutions and practicing health care professionals within the regional area of psychiatric care, patients can be assigned to an INT group from within a large district. In our clinic in Bern, some participants travel a distance of up to 60 km to their group appointments. This entails great motivation and a high level of expectation, both on the part of the patient and the patient's referrer.

Implementing intra-institutional and inter-institutional groups demands significant collaboration between the INT therapist team, the referrer (e.g. psychologists, psychiatrists, general practitioners) and the service providers. Given that it is likely that the patients do not know each other at the beginning of the treatment under such recruitment conditions, the therapists must be actively engaged in promoting a sustainable therapeutic relationship and group cohesion (► Sect. 2.5 “Motivation Building, Forming Relationships, and Group Processes”).

3.1.3 Intra-institutional Options

It is favorable for the psychotherapeutic treatment to establish INT as an intra-institutional option, for example, at an outpatient clinic or a day clinic. This ensures close interaction between the group therapists and the interdisciplinary team, and it permits integration of INT into the institution's treatment and rehabilitation concept. The specific effects of treatment on patients' everyday lives can then be further addressed between INT sessions. Since group members from the same institution are likely to know each other, building up group cohesion is substantially simplified. If any substantial prior differences exist among group members, these differences should be addressed outside the INT program.

3.1.4 Closed or Open Groups

The advantages of closed groups are obvious: each participant enters and leaves the group at the same time; each participant acquires the same amount of knowledge and coping strategies, which are practiced to the same extent. Thus, group cohesion tends to be stable. Closed groups are offered cyclically as a rule. When one group ends, the next begins. If a group has begun, subsequently referred patients are to be put on a waiting list for the following group. The closed group format is generally preferred over an open group format for patients who are able to meet for a sustained period of time.

In clinical reality however, closed groups can only be offered occasionally. This may be due to limited referral rates in small institutions or the stipulation that waitlists be avoided in order to guarantee each patient the same access to treatment within a short span of time. For these reasons, INT is also increasingly being offered as an open group. Entry and exit are possible at any time (although a certain degree of participant constancy has to be ensured for a period of time). Yet the high level of flexibility offered in an open group format has its disadvantages. It is more difficult to achieve group cohesion, and the participants are more diverse with respect to their stage of learning and insight. Also, it is harder to assess how each entry and exit affects group processes, as compared to the closed group format. As countermeasures, the therapist team might consider the adaptations to the recruitment process described in ▶ Chap. 2 (admission interview, trial session, group rules), increased session structuring compared to closed groups, or a circular repetition of therapy contents. For example, the topic of emotional perception from Module A can be recapitulated at the beginning of the introductions to social perception in Module B and to attribution in Module D. Open groups always place greater demands on the therapists when dealing with group dynamics and group processes, as compared to closed groups (▶ Sect. 3.4).

Half-open groups can also be offered as a compromise between closed and open groups. In this case, entry is only possible at certain phases, so that the group's composition remains stable within a phase. As a rule, a minimum number of treatment sessions is also determined during individual therapy planning (▶ Chap. 4). The rate of fluctuation ("drop outs") in half-open groups is lower than in open groups.

3.2 Patient Characteristics

INT is conceived for stable ambulant or day-care patients suffering from schizophrenia. The sometimes difficult content of INT's integrated intervention units is intended for more stable patients with a diagnosis of schizophrenia or schizoaffective disorder (DSM-IV-TR; ICD-10). Patients in an acute or post-acute stage of illness or chronically ill patients with significantly reduced performance levels and pronounced negative symptoms will probably be overtaxed by the interventions and content used.

Cognitive problems in the 11 cognitive target areas defined by MATRICS represent further selection criteria (Nuechterlein et al. 2004; Green et al. 2005). It should be noted that it is hardly possible to recruit persons with problems in all 11 target areas. Due to the variability of the participants' cognitive performance profiles, therapists should expect to have patients in each intervention area who exhibit differing baseline functioning. If possible, it is recommended that participants with similar baseline functioning or presenting concerns are selected for the same group.

Furthermore, inclusion of other patient populations with cognitive deficits is not recommended (e.g. patients with affective disorders with or without psychotic symptoms) since in this case the process of cognitive rehabilitation is significantly shorter than patients with schizophrenia. With the former type of patients, group processes and procedures should generally be handled differently with respect to content as well. However, it is feasible from a practical point of view for the demographic profiles of potential participants to be highly varied. For example, both younger, first episode patients and older patients of about 55 years who have had the disease for decades have successfully participated together in INT groups.

Even patients with persisting positive symptoms, but not overly pronounced negative symptoms can be accepted into INT groups. Yet if there are patients with persisting positive symptoms, therapists should make sure that their symptoms do not overly compromise their ability to be integrated into the group. INT is focused on improving and optimizing cognitive performance. The treatment of current delusional symptoms and hallucinations should be delegated to the therapist performing individual therapy. Patients with highly pronounced negative symptoms (e.g. lacking affective rapport, social withdrawal) may be overwhelmed by the group interventions. The Integrated Psychological Therapy program (IPT; Roder et al. 2008a, 2010) is more suitable for such patients (▶ Sect. 3.5.2).

3.3 Group Composition

A group size of five to eight participants has been proven to be effective. If there are more than eight participants, it becomes increasingly difficult to achieve group cohesion and to make therapeutic use of group processes. It also places excessive demands on the infrastructure. On the other hand, if there are fewer than five participants, absenteeism may make it impossible to attain the critical group size of three.

The group should be especially consistent with respect to intelligence (IQ of about 90 or higher) and diagnosis (schizophrenia or schizoaffective disorder). Patients with lower IQ and patients with brain injuries will probably be overly challenged by participation in an INT group. Furthermore, therapy content is often unsuitable for patients with a pronounced co-morbid drug abuse problem, since the problems of addiction are not addressed. On the other hand, group diversity is preferable with respect to sex and age.

Patients of a different ethnic group or nationality can only be included in the group if their language abilities are sufficient enough to understand the language-based interventions and informational materials. On-site translation by co-patients with the required language abilities is possible, but this often impedes group processes. On the other hand, patients with illiteracy problems can be supported effectively by the co-therapist and other patients.

3.4 Therapist Requirements

INT requires a highly qualified therapist team (as a rule, one primary therapist and one co-therapist). At least the primary therapist responsible for leading the group should have in-depth knowledge of the therapy's structure and methodology. The primary therapist is recommended to have completed a goal-oriented introduction workshop[1] on how to apply the four treatment modules didactically and how to vary the amount of structuring while leading a group. In addition, knowledge of group processes and group dynamics is essential. This includes the ability to lead groups and to utilize group processes therapeutically.

INT contains a number of cognitive and behavioral-therapeutic elements to be implemented within an overarching therapeutic framework. On the basis of patient-centered therapy planning, participants should be guided to engage in self-reflection and goal-oriented thinking and behaving while enhancing their ability to experience and express emotions in a situationally appropriate manner. They should also be encouraged to develop individual compensation strategies corresponding to their own life situations. Thus, INT should be understood as a psychotherapeutic method and not reduced to the term "cognitive training" as it is often referred to in Anglo-American usage. INT does indeed include an exercise component (restitution), but the goal here is not simply improvement by repeated practice. Instead, the participants learn adaptively to convert and implement acquired coping strategies. This distinguishes INT from classic, often computer-based methods of cognitive remediation. For this reason, substantial psychotherapeutic knowledge is a basic prerequisite to run an INT group successfully – knowledge that is usually acquired in postgraduate education for various professions. Completed advanced training in behavioral therapy is especially helpful.

[1] More information is available from the editors.

3.5 Differential Indication and Contrasts to IPT and WAF

INT arose as a further development to the cognitive subprograms of Integrated Psychological Therapy (IPT; Roder et al. 2008a, 2010). IPT's five subprograms integrate interventions on neurocognition, social cognition, and social competency into an overarching therapy framework (▶ Chap. 1). IPT's subprograms on social competency were further developed into specific therapy programs for the areas of living, work, and leisure (WAF, from the German "Wohnen, Arbeit, Freizeit"; Roder et al. 2008b). The question now is how to distinguish the three approaches – INT, IPT, and WAF – and which targeted patient populations are to be assigned to which programs.

3.5.1 INT

The requirements for successful application of INT discussed in this chapter can be summarized as follows: INT is especially suited for stable, ambulant or day-care patients with schizophrenia who possess deficits in various neurocognitive or social-cognitive functional areas (MATRICS). Yet this requires extensive prior clarification (supported by psychological tests, if possible) and individual therapy planning (▶ Chap. 4). Group participation should be ensured for a sustained time period. Therapists are also required to collect information regarding basic language competencies and intellectual functioning. It is recommended that patients demonstrate moderate motivation for participating in the interactive exercises and a basic level of insight into their cognitive problems. As opposed to psychoeducational approaches, the focus here is not diagnosis-based insight into the illness but rather the self-perception of cognitive functioning. Moderate persisting positive symptoms, negative symptoms (provided they are not too pronounced), and age do not represent criteria for exclusion from INT in principle, as long as they do not overly impair group processes.

So far, INT has also been applied successfully for young (first episode) patients in the prodromal phase of their illness. While some of the interventions are computer-based, they have been proven to be motivational even for older patients without any experience in using computers. Limited computer skills were not found to be a significant barrier for successful participation in INT.

INT is thus a scientifically evaluated approach for ambulant and day-care patients requiring wide-ranging cognitive remediation therapy, equipping these patients with the basic cognitive prerequisites for other specific interventions such as the treatment of social competence, cognitive therapy for persisting positive symptoms, or psychoeducation and family therapy.

3.5.2 IPT

IPT is a highly effective therapy alternative to INT for (older) patients with chronic schizophrenia and considerable functional deficits. IPT's simple, highly structured exercises on the cognitive intervention areas have a lower level of functional difficulty than INT. IPT is also less emotionally straining compared to INT. IPT has also consistently demonstrated significantly greater treatment effects on middle-aged and older patients then on control patients under standard treatment conditions (Mueller et al. 2013). The results of the research on IPT, now stretching over three decades, have also repeatedly demonstrated a reduction of negative symptoms (summarized in Roder et al. 2006a, 2011; Mueller et al. 2007; Mueller and Roder 2008). These findings were consistent with the clinical experience of many IPT users. In addition, IPT has also been successfully and effectively implemented for inpatients in the post-acute stage and for chronically ill, unmotivated and socially anxious patients. IPT, with its comprehensive, progressive sequence of subprograms for cognitive and social domains, is also recommended for patients possessing both pronounced cognitive and social deficits. IPT's social competence component comprises communication training, social skills interventions, and interpersonal problem solving. These are ideal for patients with low levels of general social competence and social integration.

3.5.3 WAF

On the basis of functional recovery (► Chap. 1), the primary therapeutic goal may lie in one of the three specific social intervention domains of residence, work, or recreation. In this case, one of the three WAF programs will be the first choice of psychotherapeutic treatment. The residential and vocational programs are specifically meant for stable and at least moderately motivated patients who can discuss individual goals for change or problems in one of the three target areas. The recreation program, on the other hand, serves to promote more active planning and use of free time. The recreational program is on a somewhat lower level of functional difficulty and emotional strain. This makes it possible to include less stable patients. Significant improvements in the area of social competence have been demonstrated for all three WAF programs (Roder et al. 2001, 2002). The patient's motivation for therapy was found to be a crucial mediator for the success of the therapy (Roder et al. 2006b; Mueller and Roder 2005). However, for a WAF intervention to be successful, existing cognitive impairments cannot hinder the acquisition of specific social skills in the three target areas. In practice, it makes good sense to implement IPT first in order to prepare less socially integrated patients for participation in a WAF program.

References

Green, M. F., Olivier, B., Crawley, J. N., Penn, D. L., & Silverstein, S. (2005). Social cognition in schizophrenia: Recommendations from the measurement and treatment research to improve cognition in schizophrenia new approaches conference. *Schizophrenia Research, 31*, 882–887.

Mueller, D. R., & Roder, V. (2005). Social skills training in recreational rehabilitation of schizophrenia patients. *American Journal of Recreational Therapy, 4*(3), 11–19.

Mueller, D. R., & Roder, V. (2008). Empirical evidence for group therapy addressing social perception in schizophrenia. In J. B. Teiford (Ed.), *Social perception: 21st century issues and challenges* (pp. 51–80). New York: Nova.

Mueller, D. R., Roder, V., & Brenner, H. D. (2007). Effektivität des Integrierten Psychologischen Therapieprogramms (IPT). Eine Meta-Analyse über 28 unabhängige Studien. *Nervenarzt, 78*(1), 62–73.

Mueller, D. R., Schmidt, S. J., & Roder, V. (2013). Integrated Psychological Therapy (IPT): Effectiveness in schizophrenia inpatient settings related to patients' age. *American Journal of Geriatric Psychiatry, 21*(3), 231–241.

Nuechterlein, K. H., Barch, D. M., Gold, J. M., Goldberg, T. E., Green, M. F., & Heaton, T. E. (2004). Identification of separable cognitive factors in schizophrenia. *Schizophrenia Research, 72*, 29–39.

Roder, V., Brenner, H. D., Müller, D., Reisch, T., Lächler, M., Zorn, P., Guggenbühl, R., Schröder, S., Christen, C., Schmidl, F., & Jenull, B. (2001). Effekte neuer kognitiv-behavioraler Therapieprogramme zur Verbesserung spezifischer sozialer Fertigkeiten bei schizophren Erkrankten: Eine kontrollierte Studie. *Nervenarzt, 72*(9), 709–716.

Roder, V., Brenner, H. D., Müller, D., Lächler, M., Zorn, P., Reisch, T., Bösch, J., Bridler, R., Christen, C., Jaspen, E., Schmidl, F., & Schwemmer, V. (2002). Development of specific social skills training programmes for schizophrenia patients: Results of a multicentre study. *Acta Psychiatrica Scandinavica, 105*, 363–371.

Roder, V., Müller, D. R., Mueser, K. T., & Brenner, H. D. (2006a). Integrated psychological therapy (IPT) for schizophrenia: Is it effective? *Schizophrenia Bulletin, 32*(Suppl 1), 81–93.

Roder, V., Müller, D. R., & Zorn, P. (2006b). Therapieverfahren zu sozialen Fertigkeiten bei schizophren Erkrankten in der Arbeitsrehabilitation. Vorteile des Aufbaus arbeitsspezifischer gegenüber unspezifischer sozialer Fertigkeiten. *Zeitschrift für Klinische Psychologie und Psychotherapie, 35*, 256–266.

Roder, V., Brenner, H.D., & Kienzle, N. (2008a). *Integriertes Psychologisches Therapieprogramm bei schizophren Erkrankten IPT* (6th, Rev. ed.). Weinheim: Beltz.

Roder, V., Zorn, P., Pfammatter, M., Andres, K., Brenner, H. D., & Müller, D. R. (2008b). *Praxishandbuch zur Verhaltenstherapeutischen Behandlung schizophren Erkrankter*, 2. Auflage. Bern: Huber.

Roder, V., Müller, D. R., Brenner, H. D., & Spaulding, W. D. (2010). *Integrated psychological therapy (IPT) for the treatment of neurocognition, social cognition, and social competencies in schizophrenia patients*. Göttingen: Hogrefe.

Roder, V., Müller, D. R., & Schmidt, S. J. (2011). Effectiveness of the integrated psychological therapy (IPT) for schizophrenia patients: a research up-date. *Schizophrenia Bulletin, 37*(Suppl. 2), 71–79.

Diagnostic Instruments, Treatment Planning, and Controlling the Treatment Process

V. Roder, S. J. Schmidt

Additional material (CD-ROM) to this book can be downloaded from http://extras.springer.com

V. Roder, D.R. Müller (eds.), *INT-Integrated Neurocognitive Therapy for Schizophrenia Patients*, DOI 10.1007/978-3-319-13245-7_4, © Springer International Publishing Switzerland 2015

In the treatment and rehabilitation of persons suffering from schizophrenia, sufficiently prepared case formulations are made for conspicuously few patients. A proper case formulation includes the following: a systematic, standardized description of resources and problems (What can the person do well? What are her everyday problems?), a diagnosis (e.g. test diagnosis, psychopathology), a case history, and a short-term, medium-term, and long-term treatment plan consistently based on these topics. A good and carefully prepared formulation of the case helps the therapist avoid early errors and minimize "trial and error" when planning treatment and rehabilitation. For example, a precise review of previous pharmacological or sociotherapeutic interventions can prevent a patient (who unsuccessfully received medication xy or occupational therapy xy 5 years ago) from being confronted with the same type of treatment again. It also does not make sense to prescribe an INT group to a patient without first evaluating his neurocognitive or social-cognitive problems and resources. A visit to an INT group should also be included when making a comprehensive treatment and rehabilitation plan. All therapists of various vocations and functions (e.g. psychologists, nurses, social workers, physicians, ergotherapists) should get together to discuss the case at regular intervals (of 6–8 weeks, for example). They can then exchange views about short-term, medium-term, and long-term treatment planning, settle on a binding procedure, or modify previous attempts. After determining these potential treatment goals, a case meeting with the patient is held. This talk takes special consideration of the desires and goals of the patient concerned ("motivation to change"). The goals established together during the discussion are recorded in writing and remain valid for the next 6–8 weeks.

The therapist leading the case prepares the information required for case formulation using the diagnostic-therapeutic process approach, which will be presented in the following brief overview.

Diagnostic-Therapeutic Process Approach

Problem Analysis

1. Unproblematic behavior and experience (resources)
2. Description of problem areas
   - (behavioral) indicators
   - cognitions
   - emotions
   - details in problem description
3. Analysis of the conditions perpetuating the problematic behavior; formulating hypotheses
   - antecedents
   - consequences
   - hypotheses
4. Analysis of motivation
   - with respect to problem areas
     - discrepancies between self-descriptions and the descriptions of others
     - patient's motivation to change
   - general
     - patient's personal (rehabilitation) goals
     - possible reinforcements
5. Current social relationships
   - intra-clinical
   - extra-clinical

Sociocultural Background

1. Development background
2. Recent changes in patient's living environment (e.g. loss of a partner or position)

Classificatory Diagnostics

1. Psychodiagnostics
2. Psychopathology (DSM-IV-TR-Diagnosis etc.)
3. Somatic findings (organic particularities they can be related to problems)

Problem/Treatment Records

1. Psychotherapeutic/sociotherapeutic methods
2. Medicinal treatment

Therapy Planning

1. Selection of therapeutic methods
2. Planning of time and content

4.1 Case Formulation: Diagnostic-Therapeutic Process Approach

In order to formulate a case using the diagnostic-therapeutic process, the responsible therapist must rely on the testimony of the patient concerned (self-description), the testimony of others (relatives, friends, caregivers), observation (provided the therapist in charge has regular contact with this patient), tests (e.g. MATRICS tests), standardized interviews (e.g. PANSS), questionnaires (e.g. ESI), and patient files (medical history).

4.2 Problem Analysis

4.2.1 Unproblematic Behavior and Experience (Resources)

As it was pointed out in ► Chap. 2, building up long-term motivation and a sustained relationship with patients with schizophrenia is a key problem. For this reason, a detailed case history is not the most important goal when making first contact with a potential INT patient and for formulating the case. Rather, a good relationship (compliance) should be established, which motivates the patient to continue coming to the therapist and to group meetings. Several sessions (five or more) should generally be planned for this. These initial sessions shape the medium-term sustainability of the therapeutic relationship. In terms of content, they focus primarily on patient resources (e.g. What can he do well? What does he enjoy?). Discussion of stressful topics should mostly be avoided. The supportive relationship offered by the therapist is characterized by interest, positive and accepting attention, and active guidance of discussion. The following discussion techniques should be avoided:

- confronting ("But you told me exactly the opposite three minutes ago.");
- mirroring (returning a patient's question back to the patient);
- silence (not saying anything);
- judging ("I think it's bad that you haven't learned a profession yet.");
- interpreting and free-associating ("You keep sliding back and forth on your chair. Are you nervous? Does our conversation remind you of a past experience? Tell me about it".; and
- asking about (negative) feelings;

As a whole, the therapeutic style at this treatment stage can be described as complementary, i.e., the patient's wishes and ideas are supplemented and supported. This data obtained directly from the patient is aggregated with other information.

After these initial sessions, the therapist-patient relationship focuses on actual problem analysis by describing the problem areas.

4.2.2 Describing Problem Areas

Exact analysis of the problem and patient behavior is a core element of the diagnostic-therapeutic process. It is needed to plan subsequent therapy and to select the right behavioral-therapeutic interventions. When creating a behavior/problem analysis, the therapist must observe the patient's behavior from several different standpoints and consider associated conditions in a systematic context. In the process, self-description and the descriptions of others serve as valuable sources of information. Yet it must be stressed that the testimony of others should often be given greater weight due to the disease pattern. It is best for the therapist in charge to start with an emphasis on resources by carefully asking the patient which of the areas already discussed might need improvement ("People can always learn more about this ... You never stop learning ... It is always possible to improve ourselves ... "). This conversation style provides many patients with a fresh opportunity to address their own problems.

The first step is to establish and describe the patient's current problems and difficulties. Each problem area is chronicled in detail and then operationalized using behavioral indicators. Also, associated cognitions and emotions are listed for each indicator. To describe the problem exactly, the frequency, intensity, and duration of certain behaviors must also be logged.

4.2.3 Analysis of the Conditions Perpetuating the Problematic Behavior; Formulating Hypotheses

This is followed by an analysis of the conditions that are perpetuating the problematic behavior. Trigger events (antecedents) should be found for every behavioral problem. These can be specific situations, cognitions, or emotional states. However, it is often impossible to find a clear antecedent for problematic behavior in the case of patients with schizophrenia. The next step is to describe the consequences of a behavior problem, both for the patient and her environment. With the knowledge of these triggering and perpetuating conditions (antecedents and consequences), it is sometimes possible to interrupt certain dysfunctional experiential and behavioral sequences – for example, in neurocognitive or social-cognitive areas with the help of INT interventions. Finally, the therapist formulates hypotheses to explain the causes of the respective problem area. These hypotheses should follow logically from behavioral indicators, cognitions, and emotions (and potentially from an analysis of external conditions as well).

4.2.4 Analysis of Motivation

A complete problem analysis also includes a careful study of motivation. As previously mentioned, motivation and willingness to cooperate – which are often low – represent fundamental problems in treating patients with schizophrenia. Patients' perceptions and those of others can differ greatly, so therapists are often faced with ethically difficult decisions when defining therapeutic goals. For this reason, motivation must be carefully analyzed. First, a comparison is made between self-description and the testimony of others. Discrepancies are ascertained by critically weighting all previously obtained data, especially hypotheses and cognitions. This occurs on two different levels: that of recognizing and describing the problem and that of attributing the cause which brought about the problem. If both levels of self-description and outside testimony are in agreement, the patient is probably motivated to change. If they do not agree, the therapist can expect low therapy motivation. In addition, the patient's motivation for therapy also depends considerably on the gravity of the problem (insight, repression, denial, etc.), on past functional experiences with solution/coping attempts, and especially on associated positive experiences with therapists and related parties. In order to include the patient's perspectives and expectations in the process of planning therapy, the therapist inquires about short-term and long-term goals (desires for change; life goals, etc.). For unmotivated patients with a low activity level, it is best to engage in specific activities that might have reinforcing value (e.g. going for a walk with somebody; being invited to have coffee together; going to the movies). Therapeutic goals are often easier to achieve with the use of reinforcements.

4.2.5 Current Social Relationships

As a further component of problem analysis, the therapist also inquires about the patient's social network. All of the patient's important social relationships within and outside the clinic must be identified. It is necessary in some circumstances to involve certain persons in the treatment process in order to enhance treatment – for example, the treatment of social cognition. Also, the roles of relevant, key contacts of a patient can be acted out in role plays by the co-therapist or other group members in the INT group, e.g., when performing exercises on attribution or theory of mind (▶ Chap. 2).

Problem analysis is supplemented with the sociocultural background, classificatory diagnosis, and by ascertaining the prehistory of the problem and previous treatment.

4.3 Sociocultural Background

By learning about a patient's sociocultural background, current difficulties and problems can be understood in the context of his or her life story. Difficulties can often arise as the result of changes in one's environment ("life events"). Only by incorporating such background information is it possible to create new experiential and learning conditions for the patient that encourage him to try out new and functional behavior patterns.

4.4 Classificatory Diagnostics

Psychodiagnosis objectifies important areas of a patient's personality and performance. It provides information about the type and level of psychotherapeutic methods to be selected. This further attunes the process of change to the patient's individual needs. Since serious impairments in cognitive functioning and social behavior are considered to be basic symptoms of schizophrenia, standardized methods are generally used to measure the level of neurocognitive and social-cognitive functioning and to determine social behavior.

◘ Tables 4.1 and 4.2 provide a selective overview of associated measurement tools.

Because the focus of this book is on cognition, the reader is referred to other sources for the (standardized) determination of social behavior (e.g. Roder et al. 2008b; ▶ Chap. 6). The exemplary ELADEB test by the team in Pomini (2011) is currently one of the most exemplary. With this test, levels of social functioning and life quality can be ascertained while taking into account the patient's individual therapeutic goals.

Data captured by standardized methods are supplemented by a description of the psychopathology and a diagnosis in accordance with ICD-10 or DSM-IV-TR. These are especially important with respect to potential pharmacological treatment. Overviews of associated measurement tools can be found in Roder et al. (2008a; ▶ Chap. 6) and elsewhere.

Finally, a careful examination of somatic findings will clarify whether certain problematic experience/behavior patterns should be attributed to organic causes.

4.5 Problem/Treatment Records

Another element in the diagnostic-therapeutic process is to establish the patient's problem/treatment records in the areas of pharmacology, psychotherapy, and sociotherapy. This can help identify recurring patterns stemming from unsuccessful therapeutic interventions to be avoided in future. In addition, the prehistory can help us trace the development of a problem under treatment conditions. In contrast to the sociocultural background of a patient, the problem's prehistory thus only plays a role with respect to past therapeutic interventions.

4.6 Therapy Planning

After the problem has been analyzed and all available data has been integrated (e.g. sociocultural background, treatment prehistory, tests, questionnaires on self-assess-

Table 4.1 Neurocognitive measurement tools

Instrument	Type	Operationalized variables
Regensburg verbal fluency test (Regensburger Wortflüssigkeitstest, RWT): Categorical and verbal fluency	Test	Speed of information processing
Number/symbol test from the Wechsler intelligence test for adults (Wechsler-Intelligenztest für Erwachsene, WIE)	Test	Speed of information processing
Trail Making Test A, TMT A	Test	Speed of information processing
Concentration-strain test, d2 (Brickenkamp 2002)	Test	Discriminative capacity under strain, sustained attention, visual scanning
Continuous Performance Test, CPT (orig. Rosvold et al. 1956; UCLA-Version: Nuechterlein and Asarnow 1992)	Computer test	Sustained attention, vigilance and impulsivity, attentional errors
Span of Apprehension Test, SPAN (UCLA version: Nuechterlein and Asarnow 1992)	Computer test	Selective attention, attention span
Color-word interference test (Farbe-Wort-Interferenztest, FWIT) (Bäumle 1985)	Test	Information processing, such as selecting, coding, and decoding in optic/verbal functional areas, processing speed
Frankfurt adaptive concentration test (Frankfurter Adaptiver Konzentrationsleistungs-Test, FAKT II) (Goldhammer and Moosbrugger 2005)	Computer test	Power of concentration, performance course
Learning and memory test (Lern- und Gedächtnistest, LGT 3) (Bäumler 1974)	Test	Retentivity, concentration, orientation
Learning aptitude and retentivity test (Lern- und Merkfähigkeitstest, LMT) (Seyfried 1990)	Test	Learning aptitude and retentivity
Standard Progressive Matrices, SPM (Raven 1971)	Test	General intelligence potential, power of observation, and clear thinking
Tower of Hanoi test (Loong 1988)	Computer test	Complex reasoning processes, abstract problem solving, procedural learning
Wisconsin Card Sorting Test, WCST (Heaton 1981)	Computer test	Flexibility of reasoning, faculty of abstraction, perseverations, concept formation
Number connection test (Zahlen-Verbindungs-Test, ZVT) (Oswald and Roth 1978)	Test	Speed of information processing

ment and the assessment of others), a therapy plan is developed. It is described in stages in terms of content and time and, in some cases, depicted graphically. Since therapy is a continuous problem-solving process, the therapy plan should be constantly checked and modified in the course of treatment. The individual intervention steps are adapted to the patient's problems, needs, resources, options, and situation (environment). Therapists should thus have exact knowledge of the patient's situation and problems as well as in-depth psychological knowledge and mastery of the basic cognitive therapeutic techniques for patients with schizophrenia. Other possible approaches can be suggested both by the patient, her reference persons, or by general conditions themselves.

The starting point of all interventions is creating a plausible model for the development and solution of the problem. Such a model accommodates the patient's need for an explanation for his problems. This "insight" is usually of critical importance for motivation during treatment. On the other hand, the model also creates transparency in the therapeutic process. Both of these aspects – consideration of patient needs and transparency in the therapeutic process – are essential conditions for the patient to assume personal responsibility for later, more efficient self-management. However, when planning treatment of persons with schizophrenia, transparency is not always possible because of the patient's (often deficient) connection with reality. In our experience, it is often difficult to explain therapeutic goals in detail so as to

4

Table 4.2 Social-cognitive measurement tools

Instrument	Type	Operationalized variables
Picture of Facial Affect, PFA (Ekman and Friesen 1976; Wölwer et al. 1996)	Computer test	Emotion perception
Face Emotion Identification Task, FEIT (Kerr and Neale 1993)	Test	Emotion perception
Bell-Lysaker Emotion Recognition Task, BLERT (Bell et al. 1997)	Test	Emotion perception
Mayer-Salovey-Caruso Emotional Intelligence Test, MSCEIT (Mayer et al. 2003)	Test and computer test	Emotion perception
Half-Profile of Nonverbal Sensitivity, PONS (Bell et al. 1979)	Test	Social perception
Social Cue Recognition Test, SCRT (Corrigan and Green 1993)	Test	Social perception
Eye/Theory-of-Mind Test, Eye-ToM (Baron-Cohen et al. 2001)	Questionnaire	Theory of Mind
Hinting task (Corcoran et al. 1995)	Test	Theory of Mind
Social Component Sequencing Task-Revised, SCST-R (Corrigan and Addis 1995; Vauth et al. 2004)	Computer test	Social schemata/ social knowledge
Ambiguous Intentions Hostility Questionnaire, AIHQ (Combs et al. 2007)	Questionnaire	Social attributions

involve the patient in every step of therapy planning. This is particularly true in cases of newly diagnosed patients or those with a very long illness duration and persisting residual symptoms. In our experience, the more serious the illness and the greater the social disintegration, the less the patient can take part in medium-term and long-term therapeutic goals and thus in therapy planning. Therapists must then make the decisions themselves, guided by ethically sound principles and responsible actions.

Concretely speaking, the particular problem areas first selected are those whose treatment seems essential to the patient. To each problem area are assigned precisely defined therapeutic methods. The next step is to determine the content and schedule of the therapy. Because of its complexity, a problem area often extends over several treatment stages, i.e., from goals that are easy to those that are more difficult. Different methods for treating cognitive behavior are used at each stage. For the sake of clarity, no more than three or four stages should be planned.

Short-term treatment goals (stage 1 or possibly stage 2) are focused primarily on motivating the patient to change. This is the only way to develop a cooperative and trusting relationship between the patient and the therapist. Then, as the treatment progresses, goals can be discussed, and possibly realized, for which the patient initially was not motivated at all, but which are important for the overall rehabilitation process for leading a more independent life. Therapeutic goals are defined in the first treatment stages only if they are realistic and can give the patient early experiences of success. The patient is involved in the planning process. Therapy content and goals are discussed with her for each intervention stage. If a stage's goals have been achieved, additional methods can be applied from the next stage to build on this achievement. If a patient is in a stage which he cannot master, the previous stage is repeated. Otherwise, the therapeutic goals and methods need to be revised.

References

Baron-Cohen, S., Wheelwright, S., Hill, J., Raste, Y., & Plumb, I. (2001). The "Reading the Mind in the Eyes" test revised version: A study with normal adults, and adults with Asperger syndrome or high-functioning autism. *Journal of Child Psychology and Psychiatry, 42*(2), 241–251.

Bäumle, G. (1985). *Farb–Wort–Interferenztest (FWIT)*. Göttingen: Hogrefe.

Bäumler, G. (1974). *Der Lern- und Gedächtnistest (LGT-3)*. Göttingen: Hogrefe.

Bell, M., Bryson, G., & Lysaker, P. (1997). Positive and negative affect recognition in schizophrenia: A comparison with substance abuse and normal control subjects. *Psychiatry Research, 73*(1–2), 73–82.

Brickenkamp R (2002) Test d2 Aufmerksamkeits-Belastungs-Test. Manual. 9., überarbeitete und neu normierte Auflage. Göttingen: Hogrefe.

Combs, D. R., Penn, D. L., Wicher, M., & Waldheter, E. (2007). The ambiguous intentions hostility questionnaire (AIHQ): A new measure for evaluating hostile social-cognitive biases in paranoia. *Cognitive Neuropsychiatry, 12*(2), 128–143.

Corcoran, R., Mercer, G., & Frith, C. D. (1995). Schizophrenia, symptomatology and social inference: investigating theory of mind in people with schizophrenia. *Schizophrenia Research, 17*(1), 5–13.

Corrigan, P. W., & Addis, I. B. (1995). The effects of cognitive complexity on a social sequencing task in schizophrenia. *Schizophrenia Research, 16*(2), 137–144.

Corrigan, P. W., & Green, M. F. (1993). Schizophrenic patients' sensitivity to social cues: The role of abstraction. *American Journal of Psychiatry, 150*(4), 589–594.

Ekman, P., & Friesen, W. V. (1976). *Pictures of facial affect*. Palo Alto: Consulting Psychologists Press.

Goldhammer, F., & Moosbrugger, H. (2005). *FAKT-II. Frankfurter Adaptiver Konzentrationsleistungs-Test. Grundlegend neu bearbeitete und neu normierte 2. Auflage des FAKT von Moosbrugger und Heyden (1997)*. Göttingen: Hogrefe.

Heaton, R. K. (1981). *Wisconsin card sorting test*. Odessa: Psychological Assessment Resources, Inc.

Kerr, S. L., & Neale, J. M. (1993). Emotion perception in schizophrenia: Specific deficit or further evidence of generalized poor performance. *Journal of Abnormal Psychology, 102*(2), 312–318.

Loong, J. (1988). *The Tower of Hanoi*. San Luis Obispo: Wang Neuropsychological Laboratory.

Mayer, J. D., Salovey, P., Caruso, D. R., & Sitarenios, G. (2003). Measuring emotional intelligence with the MSCEIT V2.0. *Emotion, 3*(1), 97–105.

Nuechterlein, K. H., & Asarnow, R. F. (1992). *Manual and computer program for the UCLA continuous performance test: Version 4*. Unpublished manual and program.

Oswald, W. D., & Roth, E. (1978). *Der Zahlen-Verbindungs-Test (ZVT)*. Göttingen: Hogrefe.

Pomini, V., Reymond, C., Golay, P., Fernandez, S., & Grasset, F. (2011). *ELADEB – Echelles lausannoises d'auto-évaluation des difficultés et des besoins*. Suisse: Unité de réhabilitation.

Raven, J. C. (1971). *Standard progressive matrices (SPM)*. London: Lewis and Co.

Roder, V., Brenner, H. D., & Kienzle, N. (2008a). *Integriertes Psychologisches Therapieprogramm bei schizophren Erkrankten (IPT)* (6th Rev. ed.). Weinheim: Beltz.

Roder, V., Zorn, P., Andres, K., Pfammatter, M., & Brenner, H. D. (2008b). *Praxishandbuch zur verhaltenstherapeutischen Behandlung schizophren Erkrankter. 2. überarbeitete Auflage*. Bern: Huber.

Rosvold, H. E., Mirsky, A. F., Sarason, I., Bransome, E. D., Jr., & Beck, L. H. (1956). A continuous performance test of brain damage. *Journal of Consulting Psychology, 20*, 343–350.

Seyfried, H. (1990). *LMT. Lern- und Merkfähigkeitstest*. Göttingen: Hogrefe.

Vauth, R., Rusch, N., Wirtz, M., & Corrigan, P. W. (2004). Does social cognition influence the relation between neurocognitive deficits and vocational functioning in schizophrenia? *Psychiatry Research, 128*(2), 155–165.

Wölwer, W., Streit, M., Polzer, U., & Gaebel, W. (1996). Facial affect recognition in the course of schizophrenia. *European Archives of Psychiatry and Clinical Neuroscience, 246*(3), 165–170.

Empirical Evidence of INT

D. R. Müller, S. J. Schmidt, V. Roder

Additional material (CD-ROM) to this book can be downloaded from http://extras.springer.com

V. Roder, D.R. Müller (eds.), *INT-Integrated Neurocognitive Therapy for Schizophrenia Patients*,
DOI 10.1007/978-3-319-13245-7_5, © Springer International Publishing Switzerland 2015

INT was evaluated in a randomized, international multicenter study in Switzerland, Germany and Austria, supported by the Swiss National Science Foundation (project number 3200 B0-108133). A total of 169 persons took part in the study. Included in the study were persons fulfilling the following criteria: diagnosis of schizophrenia or schizoaffective disorder according to ICD-10 or DSM-IV-R, outpatient or day-care treatment, age between 18 and 50, illness duration of more than 2 years, intelligence quotient of over 80 (Reduced Wechsler Intelligence Test, WIP). Grounds for exclusion included any acute psychotic episode, a primary substance dependence, or brain injury.

The 169 participants were randomly assigned to the INT group (n = 86) or to the control group (n = 83). The control group received the standard treatment (treatment as usual, TAU) without specific group therapy. The treatment phase comprised 30 sessions of 90 min each and took place twice a week over a period of 15 weeks. INT strives primarily to improve neurocognitive and social-cognitive functions and secondarily to reduce symptoms and psychosocial impairments (▶ Sect. 2.1). The test battery that was employed encompassed the basic target areas and was executed before the start of therapy (baseline, T1), after therapy (after 15 weeks, T2), and after a further 37 weeks (follow-up, T3). The colleagues involved in data collection were blind with respect to group assignments.

5.1 Results

The 169 participants had an average age of 34 years and an average illness duration of 10 years. The majority of the patients were male (69 %), single (72 %), lived alone or in a shared apartment (60 %), and worked in a protected environment (37 %). The INT and control groups did not differ significantly in terms of age, sex, education, intelligence, illness duration, current symptoms, or intake of antipsychotic medication (chlorpromazine dose equivalents).

In comparison to the control group, the INT group yielded significantly better test performances after therapy in the area of neurocognition (attention, speed of information processing, verbal memory, reasoning and problem solving) and social cognition (emotional perception and social schema). There were also significant improvements in the secondary outcome areas of negative symptoms and the level of psychosocial functioning. These treatment effects persisted over the period of 1 year (Mueller et al. 2015). Effect sizes (ES) were measured separately for the INT and the control group (Cohen 1988). After treatment, the INT group obtained small to medium ES for neurocognition (ES = 0.38) and social cognition (ES = 0.26) and large ES for negative symptoms (ES = 0.75) and the level of psychosocial functioning (ES = 0.6). These effects increased still further up to the last data collection point 1 year after the treatment commenced (ES = 0.26–1.00). ◘ Figures 5.1, 5.2, 5.3, and 5.4 show the effect sizes (ES) after therapy (T1–T2) and after 1 year (T1–T3) for all therapeutic target areas. This agrees with the results of meta-analyses, which also found that cognitive remediation therapy has stable, small to moderate effects on cognitive parameters and the level of psychosocial functioning (Mueller et al. 2007; Roder et al. 2011; Wykes et al. 2011; Kurtz and Richardson 2012).

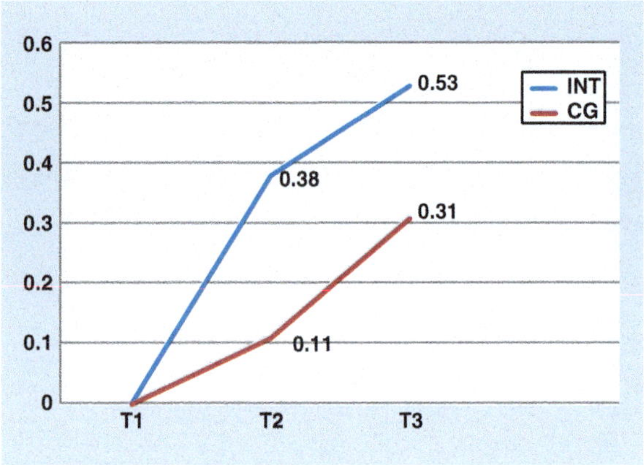

◘ **Fig. 5.1** Effect sizes (*ES*) for the area of neurocognition for the INT group and the control group (*CG*). Neurocognition: attention, speed of information processing, verbal & visual memory, working memory, reasoning & problem solving. *T1* baseline, *T2* after therapy/after 17 weeks, *T3* after 37 weeks

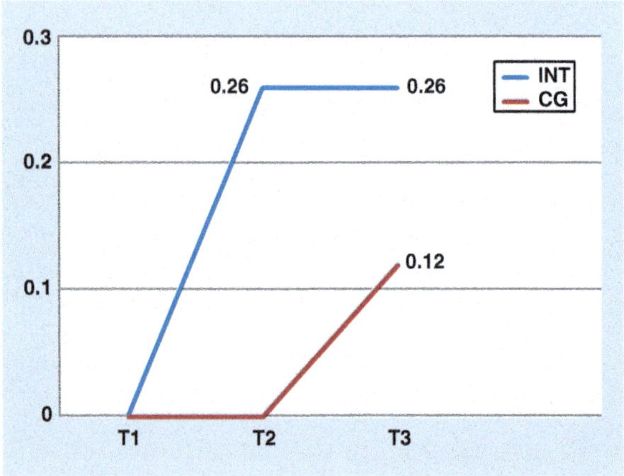

◘ **Fig. 5.2** Effect sizes (*ES*) for the area of social cognition for the INT group and the control group (*CG*). Social cognition: emotional perception, social schemata, attribution style. *T1* baseline, *T2* after therapy/after 17 weeks, *T3* after 37 weeks

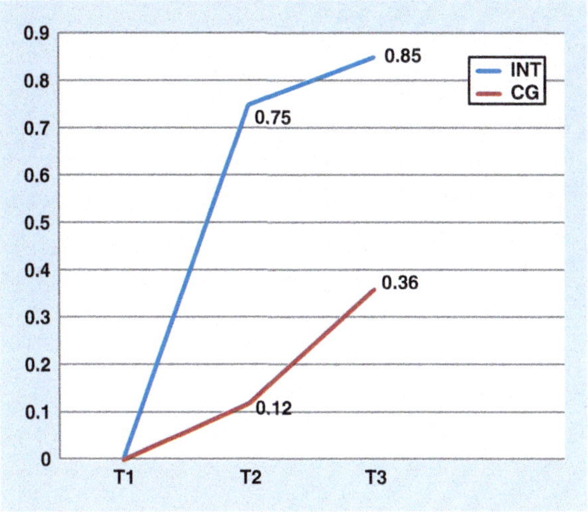

Fig. 5.3 Effect sizes (*ES*) for the area of negative symptoms for the INT group and the control group (*CG*). *T1* baseline, *T2* after therapy/after 17 weeks, *T3* after 37 weeks

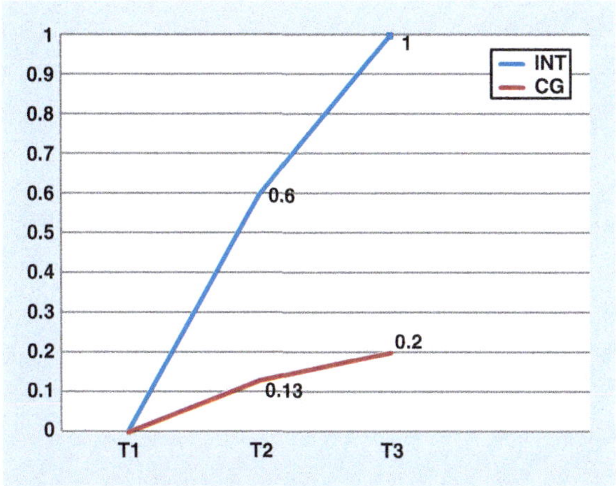

Fig. 5.4 Effect sizes (*ES*) for the level of psychosocial functioning for the INT group and the control group (CG). *T1* baseline, *T2* after therapy/after 17 weeks, *T3* after 37 weeks

In addition, the low drop-out rate of 11 % and the high participation rate of over 80 % speak for a high level of acceptance of INT by the patients (Fig. 5.1). INT is thus an integrated, evidence-based approach to cognitive rehabilitation therapy, whose cognitive effects on everyday symptoms can be statistically generalized.

Acknowledgement We would like to thank the following centers for their participation in the study: the Psychiatric Hospital of the University of Zürich (Dr. A. Theodoridou M.D.), the Biel Center of Psychiatry (Dr. A. Rausch M.D.), the University Hospital of Psychiatry in Bern, The Bielefeld Protestant Hospital, the Bethel Clinic for Psychiatry and Psychotherapy (Prof. Dr. M. Driessen M.D., C. Barenbrock, Dipl.-Psych.), the Rehabilitation Center for the Mentally Ill in Peiting-Herzogsägmühle (Dr. S. Queri, PhD; Dr. A. Gabrecht, M.D.), ARBEWE Rehabilitation Center in Nuremberg (A. Baumann, Dipl.-Psych. and G. Fisher), the Rehabilitation Center of Vitos Eltville (G. Deutschle, Dipl.-Psych); the State Hospital of Schwarzach/St. Veit (Dr. M. Keglevic M.D.).

References

Cohen, J. (1988). *Statistical power analysis for the behavioral sciences*, 2. Aufl.. Hillsdale: Lawrence Erlbaum Associates.

Kurtz, M. M., & Richardson, C. L. (2012). Social cognitive training for Schizophrenia: A meta-analytic investigation of controlled research. *Schizophrenia Bulletin, 38*(5), 1092–1104.

Mueller, D. R., Roder, V., & Brenner, H. D. (2007). Effektivität des Integrierten Psychologischen Therapieprogramms für schizophren Erkrankte. Eine Metaanalyse über 28 unabhängige Studien. *Der Nervenarzt, 78*, 62–73.

Mueller, D. R., Schmidt, S. J., Roder, V. (2015). Integrated neurocognitive therapy for schizophrenia outpatients. Effects of an international, randomized controlled trial. *Schizophrenia Bulletin*, doi:10.1093/schbul/sbu223.

Roder, V., Mueller, D. R., & Schmidt, S. J. (2011). Effectiveness of integrated psychological therapy (IPT) for schizophrenia patients: A research update. *Schizophrenia Bulletin, 27*(2), 71–79.

Wykes, T., Huddy, V., Cellard, C., McGurk, S.R. & Czobor, P. (2011). A meta-analysis of cognitive remediation for schizophrenia: Methodology and effect sizes. *American Journal of Psychiatry, 168*(5), 472–485.

Therapy Materials for the Four Treatment Areas

D. R. Müller, S. J. Schmidt, V. Roder

Additional material (CD-ROM) to this book can be downloaded from http://extras.springer.com

V. Roder, D.R. Müller (eds.), *INT-Integrated Neurocognitive Therapy for Schizophrenia Patients*, DOI 10.1007/978-3-319-13245-7_6, © Springer International Publishing Switzerland 2015

The therapy materials mentioned in ▶ Chap. 2 for the four INT treatment areas (Modules A–D) are contained on the enclosed ▶ CD-ROM. The therapy materials are organized into five tools of didactic intervention:

1. information sheets
2. worksheets
3. vignettes
4. materials
5. e-materials

The following list of intervention tools serves as an orientation aid for making printouts (Tables 6.1, 6.2, 6.3, 6.4, and 6.5). It specifies the module(s) in which the intervention tool is used as well as the number of pages to be printed. The e-materials are mainly intended to be displayed with a digital projector.

6.1 Information Sheets

Table 6.1 Information sheets

No.	Title	Module	Pages
1	Overview of the group topics and goals of INT	A	1
2	Performance and mood	A, D	1
3	How do I have more speed and concentration?	A, C	1
4	Quality of sleep and lifestyle	A, C	1
5	How can I concentrate better at work?	A, C	1
6	Filter model of perception	A, B, C	1
7	How do I recognize the feelings of others?	A, C	1
8	A gesture often says more than 1,000 words	A, C	1
9	Memory	B, C	1
10	Types of memory content	B, C	1
11	Memory tricks: inquire, repeat, and write down	B, C	1
12	Memory tricks: using the senses	B, C	1
13	Memory tricks for remembering several concepts	B, C	1
14	Memory tricks for numbers	B, C	1
15	Memory tricks for appointments or future events	B, C	2
16	Perceiving a situation	B	1
17	Assumptions are not the same as facts	B	1
18	Empathizing with others	B	1
19	Possible ways to help increase our empathy with others	B	1
20	I think, therefore I am	C	1
21	Reasoning, a matter of the brain	C	1
22	What affects our ability to reason and solve problems?	C	1
23	Difficulties reaching a goal	C	1
24	Steps for reaching a goal	C	1
25	From a complicated action to small action steps	C	1
26	How can I better find the right words?	C	1
27	Social rules and roles	C	1

Table 6.1 (*continued*) Information sheets

No.	Title	Module	Pages
28	How do I recognize that my behavior doesn't conform to rules?	C	1
29	Being able to distance ourselves: easier said than done	C	2
30	Working actively with memory	D	1
31	Costs and benefits of behavior change	D	1
32	Strategies for avoiding distraction when performing actions	D	1
33	Focusing attention	D	1
34	Distractibility during conversation	D	1
35	Is it my fault or someone else's? Looking for causes in oneself or in others	D	1
36	What can influence me in ascribing causes?	D	1
37	Vulnerability and Stress	D	1
38	How can I better control my own feelings?	D	1
39	Strategies for examining our own spontaneous causal attribution	D	1
40	Mountain hike	D	1
41	Coping with stress by yourself	D	1
42	How can I better control my own feelings?	D	1

6.2 Worksheets

Table 6.2 Worksheets

No.	Title	Module	Pages
1	How fast am I?	A	1
2	How well can I concentrate?	A	1
3	Alertness and speed/attention	A	1
4	My helpful strategies for…	A, B, C, D	1
5	Independent exercise	A, B, C, D	1
6	How well can I recognize the feelings of others?	A	1
7	How good is my memory?	B	1
8	My to-do list	B	1
9	My weekly schedule	B	1
10	Do you still remember the way?	B	13
11	How well can I recognize what is happening in a situation or a conversation?	B	1
12	How well can I reason in my everyday life?	C	1
13	How well can I solve problems?	C	1
14	My personal goal	C	1
15	Curtains up for the screen goddess; A theft in the classroom; The missing pen; Mother's purse	C	4

Table 6.2 (*continued*) Worksheets

No.	Title	Module	Pages
16	How well can I deal with social rules?	C	1
17	Which distancing strategy is good for me?	C	1
18	How well do I work with my memory in everyday life?	D	1
19	I was too distracted – I couldn't do anything!	D	1
20	Adaptability: being able to switch from one activity to another	D	1
21	How well do I understand what is happening in my daily life?	D	1
22	How well can I cope with stress? How well can I control my feelings?	D	1
23	Analyzing spontaneous causal attributions	D	1
24	Examining my causal attribution	D	1

6.3 Vignettes

Table 6.3 Vignettes

No.	Title	Module	Pages
1	One morning …	A	1
2	Later the same day …	A	1
3	And last Friday at work …	A	1
4	Rendezvous at a café	A	1
5	A day to forget	B	1
6	A telephone call for Daniel	B	1
7	Yesterday at the Italian restaurant	B	1
8	The forgotten doctor's appointment	B	1
9	Art opening	B	1
10	Back at Café Adonis	B	1
11	One film – two summaries	C	1
12	Planning the trip to the cinema	C	1
13	By bike to Café Adonis	C	1
14	Recently at the bar	D	1
15	A busy day at work	D	1
16	A truly successful day?	D	1
17	This time everything went well!	D	1

6.4 Materials

Table 6.4 Materials

No.	Title/Description	Module	Pages
1	Card-sorting exercise (IPT, Roder et al.)[a]	A, B, C	1
2	Card-sorting exercise: "Speed"	A, C, D	12
3	Card-sorting exercise: mood and concentration	A	2
4	Affect decoding stage 1: facial expressions (Ekman)[b]	A	2
5	Card-sorting exercise: emotional concept formation	A, C	9
6	Lists of words and numbers	B	5
7	Conversation examples	B	8
8	Memory conversation exercise "new identity"	B	2
9	Assessment picture series: social perception*	B	7
10	Sentences on perspective adoption	B	3
11	Group matchstick exercise	C	1
12	Exercise: place 4 or 9 cubes on a given pattern	C	22
13	Exercise: action sequences	C	30
14	10 differences between 2 pictures	D	6
15	Word search puzzle	D	3
16	Sudoku	D	6
17	Writing errors	D	3
18	Exercise: sequence of 2 categories	D	2
19	Causal attribution of events without direct interaction; given hypothesis	D	8
20	Causal attribution of events within an interaction; given hypothesis	D	8
21	Causal attribution of events within an interaction; no given hypothesis	D	11

[a]Copyright owned by the first author (available for order under roder@sunrise.ch)
[b]Copyright owned by the first author (available for order under www.paulekman.com)

6.5 e-Materials

Table 6.5 e-Materials

No.	Title/Description	Module	Pages[a]
1	Filter model: perception and memory	A	1
2	Emotion perception stage 2: facial expressions and gestures	A	10
3	Emotion perception stage 3: emotional sequences	A	3
4	Memory model	B	1
5	Remembering a route	B	24
6	Picture series on perspective adoption	B	90
7	Picture series: social scripts I	C	61
8	Picture series: social scripts II	C	19
9	Picture series: selective perception	D	9
10	Comics: social attribution	D	2

[a]Pages correspond to the number of transparencies for digital projection

Index

V. Roder, D.R. Müller (eds.), *INT-Integrated Neurocognitive Therapy for Schizophrenia Patients*,
DOI 10.1007/978-3-319-13245-7,

Index

The manufacturer's authorised representative in the EU is Springer Nature Customer Service Centre GmbH, Europaplatz 3, 69115 Heidelberg, Germany. If you have any concerns regarding our products, please contact ProductSafety@springernature.com

Printed and bound by CPI Group (UK) Ltd, Croydon, CR0 4YY
01/10/2026
02225889-0001